DIET PROOF

YOUR LIFE

DIET PROOF

YOUR LIFE

The Seven Essential Secrets of
Success

Yaël Eylat-Tanaka

Copyright

ISBN-13: 978-1518867545
ISBN-10: 1518867545
Published by: Yaël Eylat-Tanaka
Tampa, Florida
Email: dietproofyourlife@gmail.com
Blog: http://dietproofyourlife.blogspot.com
Website: http://Dietproofyourlife.net

Other Books by this Author

Diet Proof Your Life
Dreams – Poetry of the Mind
Lake of Silence
The Book of Values
Common Bits of Life
Publish Your Book Using CreateSpace
Publish Your Book on Kindle
Publish Your Book With NOOK Press
Publish Your eBook on Smashwords
Publish Your eBook on BookTango
Publish Your eBook Your Way
Revenge of the Cat Woman
SCREAMS! Three Short Stories of Terror

Acknowledgments

Many people have been instrumental in helping me create this book, from my family doctor who refused to bow to convention by giving me prescription medication, to some good friends who granted me wisdom and support. Richard Junker, Michael Thomsett and Joshua Fry, who read the manuscript and made several suggestions for revisions, deletions and inclusions.

My very special thanks to my colleagues, Dr. John E. Christ and Dr. Marcia Radke for encouraging me in this endeavor, and providing invaluable assistance in distilling complicated research into readable form.

Disclaimer

This book is meant to inspire you to take a journey of self-discovery, and thus attain a measure of serenity and self-acceptance. Nothing in this book is intended as a substitute for medical advice. Please consult your own medical professional for any personal medical issues or specific recommendations.

Table of Contents

List of Illustrations

FOREWORD

Abandon no hope ye who enter here. This is a book you cannot afford to put down. Every time you look into the mirror testifies to what you need to do for your appearance and health. There are almost too many books to count on the market portending to have the secret of losing weight and staying slim for life. The sad fact of the matter is that a diet plan may work temporarily, but cannot be sustained. The factors involved in not being able to stay the course ranges from convenience to cost. Over the years we have seen the Scarsdale, Stillman, Adkins, grapefruit, Weight Watchers, Jenny Craig and panoply of other diets strain our pocketbooks and boor our palates. There has to be a simple, logical way to manage what we eat, how we feel, and our appearance, naked and in clothes.

All life is dependent on energy to perpetuate its existence. The energy necessary for life comes from the food we eat. In nature each organism from single cell to complex plant or animal has specific requirements for maintaining its life. It is remarkable that food is consumed in the right portions and variety throughout nature. However, when it comes to humans a strange phenomenon happens: food becomes divorced from simple necessity and becomes something else. All sorts of nutrients are consumed whether beneficial or not. Harmful foods may be ingested in excess and beneficial ones not at all. How has this behavior entered into our lives and more importantly, how can we return back to what our bodies actually need?

The basic problem with eating properly rests in our head on many levels. Inside the brain there is a collection of circuits which regulate all the basic functions we take for granted, such as hunger, satiety, sleep, awareness, libido, et cetera.

Somehow the higher brain which arose to fine tune these basic circuits has interfered with the natural balance mechanism for metabolism. All around us are examples of the results of those imbalances in diabetes, obesity, cardiovascular disease, and cancer. We are in the midst of an epidemic of unrestricted overeating.

Given these basic propositions where do we go? Who can we consult without getting trite answers? It so happens, you have come to the right place. Yael Eylat-Tanaka has taken a lifetime of observation and practical eating to distill down for us a genuine method for controlling our weight without dieting. At first blush, it may seem we have heard it all before. To be sure, there are elements in common with other diet regimens. The real message is not to count calories. It is far more important to focus on how and why we eat rather than obsess on the calories. Lifestyle is paramount, as well as understanding our personal internal lives.

With a few adjustments to our thinking we can revert back to the natural order of our metabolic needs. Put the past securely where it belongs and begin to enjoy life without fear. All it takes are the steps outlined in this book. It has worked for Yael; it has worked for me; and it can certainly work for you.

John E. Christ, MD, Ph.D., Tampa, FL 2015

PREFACE

Countless books, magazines, professional journals and the media argue about the worldwide epidemic of obesity. The estimates put forth by the World Health Organization and the United Nations boggle the imagination. The world at large has become fat, with the largest incidence of obesity found in the United States. Consider that the average weight of an adult human anywhere in the world is 137 pounds; but the average weight for an adult in America is 178 pounds! To make matters worse, the statistics point to even more frightening data: White North Americans make up only 6 percent of the world population, yet account for a whopping 34 percent of the incidence of obesity. Put another way: fully 34 percent of the world's obesity cases are right here in the United States. If that is not shocking enough, compare those rates to Asia, with some 61 percent of the world population, yet only 13 percent of its weight is due to obesity.

These figures should astonish us all. The irony is that these figures apply to the richest country in the world, the most developed, scientifically advanced, and leading the world rates of obesity and diabetes and their attendant consequences.

This is not a diet book - there are enough of those on the market. Anything from low-fat to high-carbohydrate, diet shakes, paleo, and meat-lovers diets — all are represented with varying degrees of technical explanations, and often a mind-boggling array of menus and recipes. Whether these diets are effective or not is not the issue here. There is a great deal of research pointing to the fact that weight-loss diets do not work because they require an individual to restrict food intake to the point where the body thinks it is in starvation mode. On the other hand, all diets do work if their principles and concepts are adhered to. Indeed, this is the crux of the matter: Diets do work if you work them. There is no mystery here. So what's the problem? The problem is that "working" a diet, staying on a regimen of any kind is inordinately difficult, especially if it represents a departure from one's familiar habits.

But it can be done. Whether you wish to shed body weight for health reasons or merely cosmetic; whether your doctor has admonished you that you are critically endangering your health; or whether you wish to beef up your biceps and abdominals for the next Mr. Universe competition, the predicament is the same: how to stick to a diet.

The countless diet books on the market seem to have one thing in common: They all trumpet their programs as fast and easy. As you leaf through a few promising books at the bookstore, you settle upon those that seem to resonate with your own ideas, and embark on their program full of enthusiasm and gusto, only to find yourself a day or two later dragging your feet, frustrated, tired, and ready to abandon all efforts and raid the refrigerator. Sound familiar?

This book attempts to address those internal conflicts by providing encouragement and understanding of the process, thus bolstering your resolve. You will not discover a magic bullet here; but you may discover yourself.

Yaël Eylat-Tanaka, Tampa, FL 2015

INTRODUCTION

This is a chronicle of my journey of self-discovery. To that end, I have discovered certain essential elements to living life fully and gracefully, confronting its challenges, and remaining centered and balanced through them all. In this book, I discuss seven such elements that I believe promote healthy living, though certainly there are many more that might fit into the model. Indeed, all these elements are interconnected and dovetail one into the other to promote and sustain a life that is rich, happy, and healthy, a life of joy for oneself and those around us.

Come on this journey with me. I will share my experiences and the discoveries I have made along the way, and in so doing, hopefully inspire you to discover your own inner beauty and strength.

The day I stepped on the scale and registered 40 pounds above my so-called optimal weight, I swore I would never eat again. It was panic run amuck, and of course, my "resolution" did not last. I wanted to hide -- from the world, from my colleagues at work, even from my husband. I assiduously avoided looking at myself in the mirror. I cried. I became depressed and anxious. I felt overwhelmed. I did not know how to proceed, whether to embark on yet another extreme diet advertised to elicit loss of 14 pounds in two days, or seek the services of a sympathetic shrink. Obsessively, I stepped on the scale again for confirmation. The results were the same: FAT. What was I going to do? How do I cancel that information? How do I go back in time, before I knew about it; when I could somehow delude myself that my overeating did not matter? Or that water retention made my clothes feel too tight?

I tried to rationalize that I was not clinically obese. Flabby and deconditioned, yes. But then, I reasoned, anyone who weighs more than 85 pounds nowadays is considered fat. It didn't work. I felt unattractive, definitely not a reflection of today's "norms" as promulgated by the media, with the single-minded obsession with thinness that we have in our culture.

In those days, Fen-Phen (the anti-obesity combination drug fenfluramine/phentermine) was very popular, so I made an appointment with my doctor. I wanted to take the easy road. Take a pill and wake up thin the next morning. As the doctor came into the examining room, I blurted out, "I'm desperate to lose 20 pounds!" His answer was swift and dry: "Not with Fen-Phen, you're not" Oh, my gosh! He knew why I was there! He anticipated me, and cut me off at the pass. I was crushed. Worse, I began to feel truly desperate. My last hope for a quick fix was gone.

The pattern was so familiar: full of enthusiasm and resolve the first day, only to have my fervor dissipate that very afternoon with the first hunger pangs. If I succeeded in keeping to a low-calorie diet through that evening, I was almost certain to abandon all efforts by the following day. I was convinced that without some outside source in the form of an appetite suppressant, I was doomed to keep my excess weight forever, along with the depression that accompanied it, the self-consciousness, and the defeat I felt at not being able to take control. The good doctor then added rhetorically, "And what will you do after you stop taking the pills? You can't take them for the rest of your life. Besides, they can cause irreversible pulmonary hypertension. You'd be better off talking to a psychologist." Pulmonary hypertension? Irreversible? With my history of asthma, that was not good.

Much as I wanted that crutch, I knew in the deepest crevices of my being that he was speaking an inalienable truth: I could not take pills forever, and whatever excess weight I was carrying was a *symptom* of something much deeper that I needed to understand. As dejected as I felt at not being "supported" by the doctor, I began to realize that the only way to overcome my sense of defeat would be to shift my focus from fighting my weight to one of acceptance and responsibility. The task was mine to grapple with, and mine to discover a solution to.

As I drove home, I suddenly became serene for the first time. My focus had to shift from losing weight to accepting myself as I was. I had to accept that learning self-control over my eating would likely be a challenge. I might even fail. Given my vast experience in the field, I almost expected to fail. Yet I knew that my goal had to shift.

I therefore endeavored to learn all I could about myself: What were the triggers that drove me to overeat; why was I using food to deal with my feelings; indeed, why was I unacceptable to myself just as I was – chubby, but still quite a good human specimen. I was smart, fastidious, energetic, and had quite a few good qualities. Surely, I could put some of my attributes to good use.

At that moment I surrendered. I would learn to take care of myself, discovering my pains, healing the hurt, and learning to face life without a crutch. I read books, talked to friends, saw a psychologist, meditated. I began to write about my feelings, and resolved to remain aware when I had cravings, so as to analyze what was behind them, what was the trigger that precipitated them. I began to explore why I was gravitating to particular foods.

I read all I could on nutrition. *Food and Mood* by Elizabeth Somer became my bible. I was determined to avoid obsessive calorie counting and deprivation. I was not going to start another reducing diet, because a diet implied something temporary, with a beginning and an end, and the eventual return to eating "normally." That had not worked before, and I came to accept that what I needed was a lifestyle change, not a quick fix.

I had tried gimmicks, tricks, weight loss programs, and support groups. All of them worked to the extent that their program was sound, but I did not stay with any of them for very long. They were all temporary, until I learned a few essentials that would become my guides. I realized then that weight loss in itself was not the goal. There were other issues I was struggling with, and I could not make weight loss my only focus. Any weight that I lost would have to occur as part of a larger plan. This book is the distillation of the discoveries I made.

I already knew that in order to lose weight, I needed to eat less. The proliferation of diet books that come on the market each year attest to the fact that we are all looking for an easier way to be slim through some trick or gimmick, anything that will ease the task.

I have often mused that I want to be thin without going through the pain, deprivation and aggravation of a diet. I want it to simply "happen." I want to make some kind of commitment to losing weight, and for that weight to magically disappear, without having to pay my dues. While this statement may sound absurdly simplistic, in truth, losing weight *is* simple. It is simply a matter of taking in less food than one needs. However, the implementation and compliance are much more difficult to implement, and there's the rub.

Through writing and meditation, I came to realize that my life was very stressful. I worked long hours at a home business, and had few hobbies and fewer friends. I resolved to identify the stresses, and attempt to reverse or eliminate them. I enjoyed my work, so that was not a source of stress. But spending hours at my computer might be creating stress of which I might not be aware. I did not have regular mealtimes, and by the time my work had released its emergency grip, it was typically 4 o'clock in the afternoon. By that time, I was ravenous, and would eat indiscriminately, both in type of food and amount. All I wanted was relief.

My efforts involved writing exercises designed to learn about myself. I began to make lists of things I enjoyed and had missed for lack of time. For example, I love colors, sunshine and music, especially classical music, and yet, my waking moments were consumed by computer work. Something was amiss.

My first step then was to sign up for watercolor classes. Simultaneously, I began to study voice. I figured these pursuits could mitigate whatever stress I was experiencing. Here were two activities that I enjoyed, which could enhance my life, and could have only positive effects on me.

My journaling continued. I deliberately did not obsess about making entries every single day. I instinctively knew that whatever recovery I was to enjoy, would have to come gently, without forcing it, without obsessing about it. I had to commit to change, and then surrender. The following is frequently misattributed to Johann Wolfgang von Goethe, but was actually quoted by William Murray:

"Until one is committed, there is hesitancy, the chance to draw back-- Concerning all acts of initiative (and creation), there is one elementary truth that ignorance of which kills countless ideas and splendid plans: that the moment one definitely commits oneself f, then Providence moves too. All sorts of things occur to help one that would never otherwise have occurred. A whole stream of events issues from the decision, raising in one's favor all manner of unforeseen incidents and meetings and material assistance, which no man could have dreamed would have come his way. Whatever you can do, or dream you can do, begin it. Boldness has genius, power, and magic in it. Begin it now."

William H. Murray

Seventeen years have passed since then. The weight came off, but more importantly, I have learned that my weight is simply a reflection of my lifestyle; and my lifestyle is one of my own making. I discovered some compelling principles to live by, applicable to everything from how to manage my eating to how to manage life itself. Read through them, assimilate them, and see if any of them ring true. If they do, adopt them, include them in your life; if not, simply discard them. We are all individuals, and what may be true for one may not apply to another.

WHY DIETS FAIL

- ➤ The Irony of Abundance
- ➤ Sugar Not So Sweet
- ➤ The Typical American Diet
- ➤ The Costs of Obesity
- ➤ The Effects of Obesity
- ➤ Your Brain on a Diet

WHY DIETS FAIL

There is a dichotomy between the food industry's pecuniary interests and the government's attempts to reduce the incidence of obesity and its related diseases. Over the past 40 years or so, the food industry has provided us with no-sugar, no-fat and no-carb alternatives to common foods, yet, the overwhelming data indicates that we have been getting fatter despite those efforts. This is partly because any efforts to eliminate one ingredient results in overcompensating with another: sugar-free cookies contain just as many calories as regular cookies because of the added fats and other chemicals used to make the cookie palatable. Reduced fat food items are supplemented with extra sugar or salt for the same reason.

Also, our lifestyles have become overscheduled. We are busier than ever, with both parents working outside the home, and children are involved in a myriad of extracurricular activities. This is where fast food has become a godsend. No one has time to cook anymore. With the proliferation of restaurants serving gigantic portions of food at reasonable prices, our kitchens have become extensions of our living rooms, but not the hearth from which to prepare healthful meals shared with family. The Norman Rockwell paintings are of a lifestyle long ago forgotten. We are being fed conflicting information: We are admonished of the dangers of obesity, heart disease and diabetes while simultaneously being exposed to commercials extolling the dubious virtues of any number of processed foods! Is it any wonder we are confused?

One crucial characteristic of our diet nowadays is that it is processed. No matter how the food industry tries to remake its offerings, most of the foodstuff we purchase in grocery stores is refined or otherwise processed. Indeed, the food we buy and consume is not only processed, it also contains inordinate amounts of additives to extend its shelf life. Even commercials that depict food freshly grilled before our eyes has been processed, injected with preservatives or antibiotics, or freeze-dried prior to shipment. French fries are freeze-dried, dusted with flour and other preservatives before being shipped in enormous heaps to various eating establishments. Hamburgers, cold cuts, pasta, cheese, pizza - almost everything we eat has been processed. It is rare to find food in its natural state.

Curiously, in yet another ironic twist, a great deal of media attention is given on encouraging people to eat their vegetables. But this suggestion is presented in a rather unappetizing manner: steamed carrots or peas, without added flavoring of any type, and without taste. No wonder people avoid them! It is hardly surprising to see those very commercials showing actors turning their noses up or children sneaking the broccoli to the dog under the table. In response to the growing obesity epidemic in the United States, steaming has become the recipe du jour. To be sure, the steaming method does conserve vitamins and minerals, but if people won't eat them, all their touted health benefits are useless. The government's attempts to encourage a reduction in saturated fat, sugar and salt in people's diets has paradoxically managed to squash any desire to eat those very foods which support good health.

The Irony of Abundance

We are surrounded by abundance; we are bombarded with advertisements that tantalize our taste buds; we live harried lives, which make it all too easy for us to resort to fast-food. We no longer have to forage for our food – it is easily available everywhere, and for the most part, is relatively cheap. Our incomes are sufficient to permit us a life of relative plenty. And yet, with all the scientific advances in health, proper nutrition and the scourge of obesity, as a society, we find ourselves getting fatter every year, battling an ever-growing epidemic of obesity-related diseases, and being less and less in control of our health, especially as it relates to weight. There are thousands of weight-loss books, websites, 12-Step programs, TV programs that provide healthy recipes, and companies that, for a fee, will deliver the "proper" foods directly to our doorstep. Billions of dollars are spent on weight loss efforts throughout the world. Yet we keep getting fatter.

What's the problem? The problem is one is inconsistency, which leads to confusion.

The problem also rests squarely with the very abundance we enjoy. We simply have too many choices, and food has become a source of entertainment, rather than sustenance. Consider our ancestors. They lived in caves, enjoyed little protection from predators, including competing tribes, and foraged for roots, tubers and fruit, with the occasional wild animal that might sustain their clan for a week or two, if they were lucky enough to know how to protect their kill from hyenas and other hungry marauders. Their diet was meager and unpredictable. Their diet was characterized by mostly plant foods, a little animal protein, fish for those who lived close to the ocean, and very little fat.

As society progressed, farming began to gain hold, and grain became a staple in the diet. In addition to grains, other plant foods continued to dominate the diet, along with occasional eggs, milk and cheese from the goals and sheep, and the rare lamb or goat that would be slaughtered on special occasions.

The quantity of food was still limited, and sources of dietary fat were quite limited. It would be many years before sugar made its appearance as a dietary ingredient.

The Industrial Revolution saw the burgeoning of a society that moved from the farm to the city, and that move was, in fact, revolutionary. Now people worked for a wage; they worked outside the home, and in many cases, worked increasingly sedentary jobs. As the farm lay fallow, the physical effort needed for tilling and planting, harvesting and storing of food was no longer necessary, and along with this abrupt diminishment in physical activity came a concomitant reduction in our caloric needs. Said another way, less food was needed.

The Industrial Revolution also brought with it technological innovations, including the latest kitchen appliances that made work easier, and the ability to process food on an industrial level, making many foods heretofore scarce much more easily available. Sugar, coffee, cocoa, flour. Our staple grains were now being processed by fancy machines. In short order, we began to learn how to separate the chaff from the germ of the seeds, and what we produced was this wonderful pure white powder that we now know as flour. It was a novelty at the turn of the century. With increasing affluence and upward mobility, society wanted to enjoy the fruits of these innovations, and it became fashionable to bake little white cakes with sugar icing to be served on special occasions.

The kind of foods we enjoyed for thousands of years has become distorted and manipulated into processed and bioengineered fare that we consume without a second thought. We feed our babies manufactured foods; and we gladly support the restaurants and supermarkets that sell them. What has sustained us for thousands of years has now come gushing forth by leaps and bounds in the span of just a few generations. The Industrial Revolution began in the middle of the 18ᵗʰ Century, and by the turn of the 20ᵗʰ Century, has witnessed a complete shift in our lifestyles, along with ever-expanding waistlines. The graph below shows the rate of obesity from 1962 to the present, in males and females, ages 20-74. In 1962, obesity rates for this wide age group averaged 13 percent, but by 2010 had risen to a staggering 35.9 percent of 20-74 year-olds, and is projected to be 50 percent by 2030. If we continue in this vein, it is anticipated that by the turn of the next century, obesity rates will be 100%.

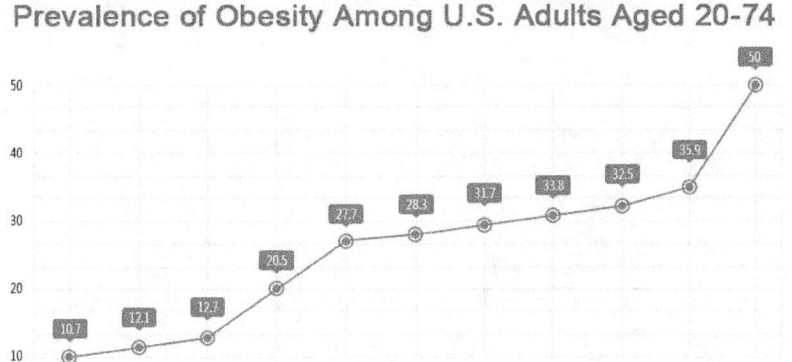

Prevalence of Obesity Among U.S. Adults Aged 20-74

What is even more astounding is that the worst incidence of obesity is right here in the good old United States.

The chart on the following page displays obesity rates in selected countries, with the United States prominently placing in first place. That is a dubious honor!

It is clear that obesity is on the rise worldwide, but how did we get to this point? We shall explore the various causes and effects of obesity in the following sections.

13

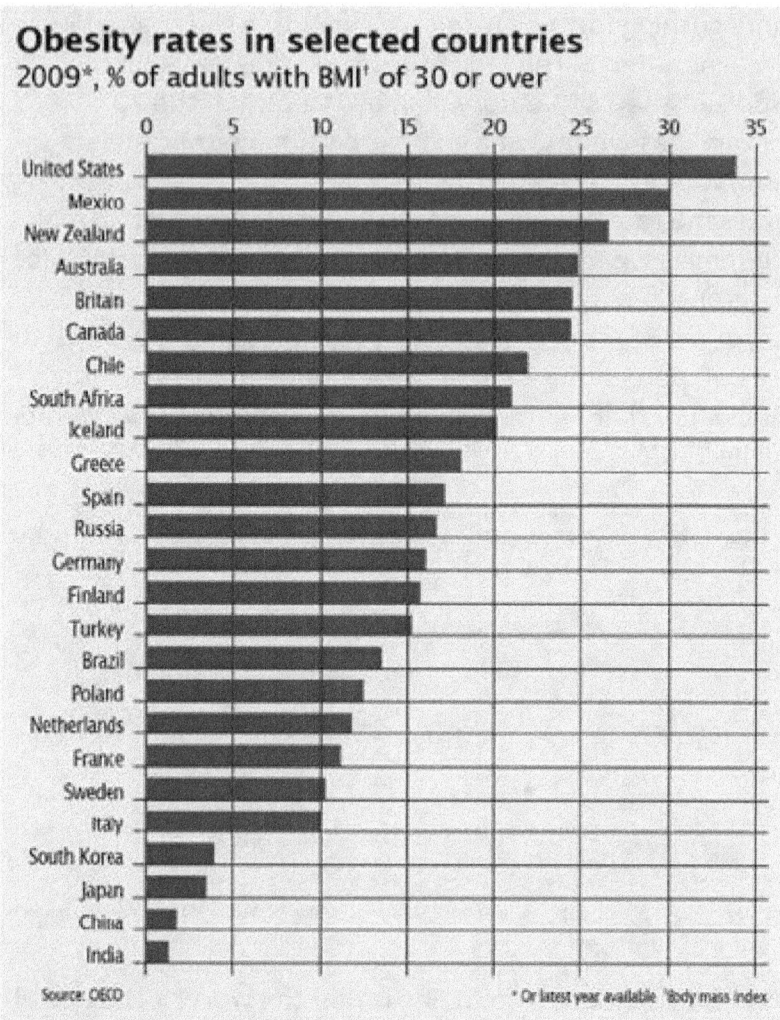

Obesity rates in selected countries
2009*, % of adults with BMI' of 30 or over

Source: OECD

* Or latest year available   'Body mass index

Adapted from *The Economist*, September 23, 2010.

Sugar Not So Sweet

For political reasons, the sugar industry has been favored by the government for generations. Sugar in its many forms serves several functions, not the least of which is increasing palatability of food, as well as increasing its shelf life. Some of our most hallowed business concerns include the beverage industry, with sales of popular sodas, juice drinks, power drinks, sports drinks and flavored waters consuming huge shelf real estate in our supermarkets. Each can of soda can pack up to 190 calories and contain as many as 12 teaspoons of sugar! That's enormous when considering that the human body does not require refined sugar at all for health. Some studies estimate that the average American consumes between 150 and 180 *pounds* of sugar per year! One hundred years ago, we consumed fewer than four pounds of sugar per year. What happened to cause such dramatic change?

In a word, we became more affluent – and busier.

Before the Industrial Revolution, when people worked the farms to grow their food, and the corner general store was the place to purchase goods, life was harsh and food was difficult to obtain. Technology consisted of pushing an ox and tiller, spending hours sowing and reaping, milking the cows, then husking the corn and preparing meals. In time, as industry began to expand, it became a luxury to bake little white cakes with white sugar and white flour to serve our guests. It was a badge of the rich.

Since then, our lives have evolved to become dependent on more and more technology, with increasingly busy schedules, leading to the ubiquitous fast food habit. But as our food has become easier to obtain, it also became less expensive, faster, and sadly, less nutritious.

Nowadays, much of the food consumed is processed. Processed food is that which has been altered from its natural state (more on that below). Food has been manipulated, mixed with foreign ingredients, such as coloring and flavoring, in some instances biologically engineered, and processed with added salt, sugar and fat to increase shelf life and palatability. Indeed, there are some who believe our food is specifically processed to be addictive.

One of the main ingredients used to process food is sugar. Sugar in its many forms appears on almost every food we eat. Consider the following list:

- Candy
- Cakes
- Bread
- Puddings
- Ice Cream
- Doughnuts
- Ketchup
- Canned vegetables
- Frozen meals
- Hot dogs
- Peanut butter
- Pickles
- Crackers
- Pizza
- ...and many others.

Consider the following chart showing the increase in our sugar consumption over the last 300 years. Granted that 300 years seems like a very long time, but the rising slope showing the increase is quite steep, signifying that our sugar consumption has risen exponentially, especially since the 1900s, when we consumed about 90 pounds of sugar per year and that has now doubled:

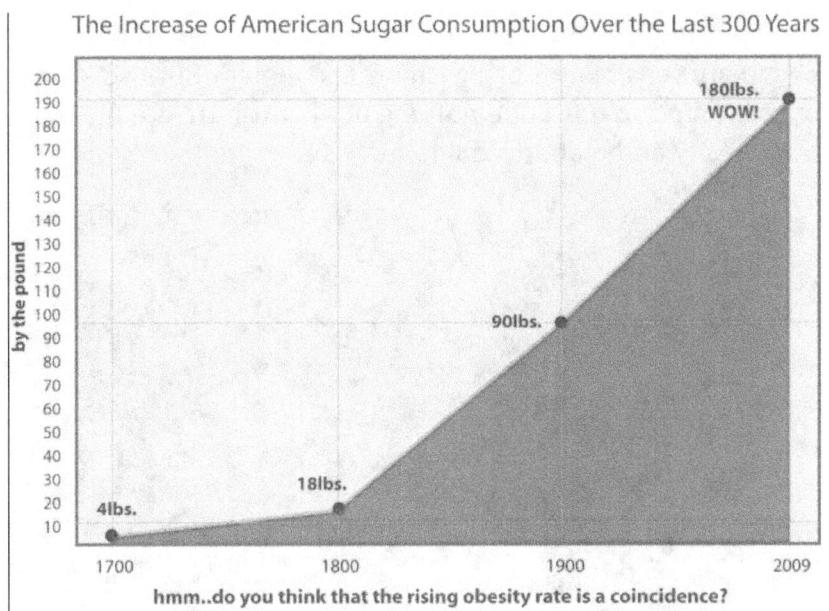

The Increase of American Sugar Consumption Over the Last 300 Years

hmm..do you think that the rising obesity rate is a coincidence?

We are now consuming on average 180 pounds of sugar per year!

The Typical American Diet

The American consumer has been raised on television and commercials, many about food. Quirky and often cute ads appear depicting a happy family quarreling over toaster waffles; or a child who is served a favorite macaroni and cheese plate by a smiling mother; an infant being fed pudding by its doting grandmother; barbecue commercials with all manner of subliminal messages evoking the free and rugged lifestyle of the cowboy – and many, many other such messages, all designed to seduce us into consumption.

Indeed, that seduction is carried forth by the restaurants as well. The food service industry is in hard competition for our dollars. They compete with individual portions that would serve a family of four in other parts of the world, with coupons and free meals that are designed to appeal to the pecuniary sensibilities of the smart consumer. But this kind of consumption has done nothing but contribute greatly to our obesity and diabetes epidemic.

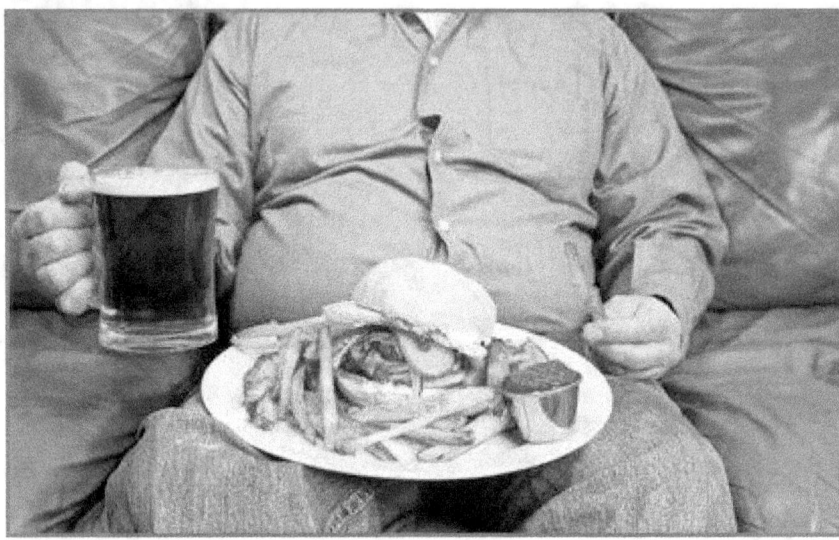

A meal of hamburger with all the fixins', French fries and a beer is as American as apple pie! The expression itself exemplifies the trouble we have created for ourselves! The advertising industry has created clever ways to lull us into accepting misinformation, and we blithely follow their recommendations. Instead of doing our own research, we fall back lackadaisically and assent to the wisdom of the "professionals." We believe the media when they promote absurd concepts such as canned pasta being "good for you." A popular commercial depicts a mother shopping with her child, passing an array of Chef Boyardee canned ravioli, and the saleslady almost blurting out that there is a full serving of vegetables in every bowl, but is thwarted by the concerned mother who worries that her child will not eat it if he knew he was consuming vegetables! And we accept such drivel as cute!

Later in this book, under the chapter on the Mediterranean diet, I discuss the incredible variety and rich flavors of vegetables of every kind. Indeed, the Mediterranean diet is legendary in its healthfulness and variety.

The Costs of Obesity

Obesity is a far more serious condition than being an esthetic concern. Obesity is expensive. The obvious costs directly related to obesity include the enormous expenditures on diets, drugs, weight loss clinics, bariatric surgery, etc., as well as the medical costs associated with obesity-related diseases, such as cardiovascular disease, stroke, cancers, diabetes, hypertension, Alzheimer's disease, to name just a few. But what about the indirect costs of obesity? High rates of absenteeism from work results in lost wages to the employee and lost production to the employer. Insurance is far more costly for the obese, covering both the costs of treating obesity and its related illnesses, as well as long-term disability payments. By some estimates, the United States spends roughly 21 percent of its healthcare funds on obesity-related ailments, this according to a study conducted by the Harvard School of Public Health Obesity Prevention (table below), versus the other representative countries in the table that spend a fraction of that.

A Snapshot of Obesity-Related Costs [1,2]

Country	Obesity-Related Costs (% of total spending on health care)	Publication Year
Brazil	3.0–5.8	2007
China	3.4	2008
Canada	2.9	2001
France	0.7–1.5	2000
Japan	3.2	2007
Sweden	2.3	2005
U.S.	20.6	2012

This is an extraordinary sum. This is comparable to a family with an annual income of $60,000, spending $12,600 of its after-tax budget on obesity and its related problems. This is over $1,000 per month! Over a lifetime, that sum is magnified manifold.

Other sources give the costs as topping $300 billion annually, when considering intangibles such as low productivity, absenteeism, obesity counseling, premature death, bariatric surgery, and rehabilitation (Pianin & Ehley). The obesity epidemic has extremely far-reaching consequences in terms of the very survival of our society.

Taking a different tack, imagine how much money you could save by avoiding obesity, taking preventive measures to protect your health, which is your greatest asset. Say a conservative estimate for direct and indirect costs of major degenerative diseases in later life is $500,000. Now imagine you exercise a mere 30 minutes a day for 50 years, as recommended by numerous experts, including Dr. Mehmet Oz and Dr. Deepak Chopra. That's about 180 hours a year, or 9000 hours during your adult lifetime, from age 20 to 70. At a "savings" of $500,000, that works out to $55 an hour. How much do you earn at your current job?

The Effects of Obesity

The media as a whole glibly broadcasts the increasing incidence and dire consequences of diabetes through a commercial lens, with innumerable commercials about new drugs come on the market to reduce blood sugar, or eliminate foot pain and tingling. The drug companies rake in millions of dollars to develop new compounds, as doctors and

20

hospitals pad their respective bottom lines with the victims of diabetes. Indeed, an entire industry has sprung up around an epidemic that is of our own making.

It is no secret that diabetes has become epidemic in the United States. But that is a misconstrued focus. To be sure, diabetes is a grave chronic disease that has assumed epidemic proportions in the United States, but the underlying problem is obesity. We have become affluent. Ours is a capitalistic society where financial profit is of paramount importance to industry as a whole. The food industry, the sugar industry, the restaurants and fast food concerns all vie for our dollars. The competition is fierce, and as consumers we gravitate to the best value for our dollars. All-you-can-eat buffets litter every street corner, ice cream and cupcake specialty cafes sprinkle the landscape, and television commercials tout the pleasures of chips, dips and bonbons. Is it any wonder we have become a nation of giants?

The effects of obesity are far-reaching indeed. From unsightly blubber to joint pain, obesity and overweight have taken their toll. Orthopedists are called upon to replace joints, while rehabilitation centers abound to get us back on our feet after surgery. Heart disease is rampant because of the increased stress of excess fat on the heart. Many kinds of cancers, from colon and breast cancer, form as a direct result of obesity. Breathing and circulation problems are linked to obesity. Pregnancy and delivery suffer as a result of obesity, not to mention problems conceiving. Kidney problems, fatty liver and gallbladder disease, diabetes and stroke all are directly linked to obesity. The effects of obesity on society are staggering in terms of health, productivity, social and emotional health of its citizens, healthcare costs and even national defense. According to research conducted at the Harvard School of Public health, obesity is second only to tobacco as the cause of death in the United States, but while smoking rates are decreasing, obesity and its related maladies are on the rise.

Your Brain On A Diet

The human species evolved during a time of scarcity. Food was unpredictably available, so our bodies learned to adapt to such scarcity. More precisely, it was the limbic system in our brains that evolved to help us survive our fragile existence. Over millions of years, we survived by devising a biological system to conserve energy. Until relatively recently in evolutionary terms, our existence was hand-to-mouth. Yet in the blink of an eye, humanity was faced with overabundance.

Around the end of the nineteenth century, beginning of the twentieth, our lifestyles morphed from agriculture to industrial. For the first time, society began to move away from the farms, where food and goods were produced, to the cities where our labors were now exchanged for a salary. Our food, goods and services were now exchanged for money. But there are sometimes negative consequences to progress. Where people no longer needed to get up in the wee hours to milk the cows or tend the crops, they now were able to purchase food at the market. In time, more crops became available to the masses, at lower costs, and famine was no longer an issue. Food was available; food was plentiful; and scarcity was a vestige of our primitive ancestry.

The problem is that where society has progressed by leaps and bounds, our biology has not. Our brains have remained primitive.

Are you surprised? Have we not evolved since the first creatures walked out of the primordial soup? Have we not become bigger and stronger, better able to sustain the ravages of illness and deprivation? Have we not seen an end to scourges and famine?

True, we have. We have conquered diseases that used to decimate entire populations; we have wiped out many health threats; we have built dams and harnessed clean water; we have learned how to grow crops and distribute them worldwide. But we have not succeeded in changing our biology. Indeed, that has never been a priority.

We have made huge advances, some very rapidly, without concern for the effect that some of our advances fly in the face of good health. For example, for all our advances in technological convenience, we have designed a life where almost everything we do is sedentary. We drive everywhere, we take elevators, and then sit at desk jobs for hours. At the end of our work day, we then return home only to wolf down some fast food then resume our sedentary state by sitting in front of our television sets. We snack on salty crackers or ice cream, drink beer and repeat the entire experience the following day.

The limbic system is a complex network of nerves near the cortex of the brain that is concerned with instinct and mood. It controls the basic emotions such as fear or anger, as well as our drives for sex, hunger or protection of our young. The limbic system is the most primitive part of the brain. It is the pleasure center, and plays a critical role in sexual arousal and the pleasurable feelings evoked by addictive drugs. Importantly, it is also involved in the pleasure we get from certain foods, especially refined sugars and carbohydrates. This is an abbreviated definition for what is arguably the most important element contributing to our current battle of the bulge. In short, we are set on cruise control by our very hormones! We are designed to gorge in order to forestall starvation in times of scarcity. Our brains are physiologically designed to conserve energy for the purposes of survival. That means increasing the heart rate and flow of adrenalin when danger is imminent, or slowing down the metabolism when food is scarce, all in an effort to ensure survival. The limbic system functions independently from our conscious control. The problem is that our bodies, or more specifically our brains, have not adapted to a world of plenty: We no longer live in caves; we no longer have saber-tooth tigers nipping at our heels; we no longer have to dig for roots or hunt animals for our meals. Most importantly, we no longer suffer food scarcity. Yet our brain has not yet caught up. We have not kept pace with the evolution of technology.

We have advanced by enormous strides in a mere one hundred fifty years or so, reversing lifestyles that had sustained us for millennia. While technology moves forward at breakneck speeds, our brains are still mired in primitive survival mode, and these survival mechanisms urge us to gorge on as much food as possible. And the food industry obliges!

Therefore, our prime task is to try to override our natural instincts with some unnatural conscious self-control, until our brain catches up with our current milieu. This is not likely to happen in our lifetimes. But exerting self-control on our instincts by drastic deprivation will simply not work: As soon as the brain detects even a hint of scarcity, it will work overtime to compensate – ergo, the binge.

Your brain on a diet spells revolt. Not only do diets not work, they are biologically impossible.

Let us turn our attention to what we can do to anticipate brain rebellion while we try to avert obesity and maintain good health. The following are seven essential secrets that are particularly helpful in our quest to override our natural tendencies.

THE SEVEN
ESSENTIAL SECRETS
OF SUCCESS

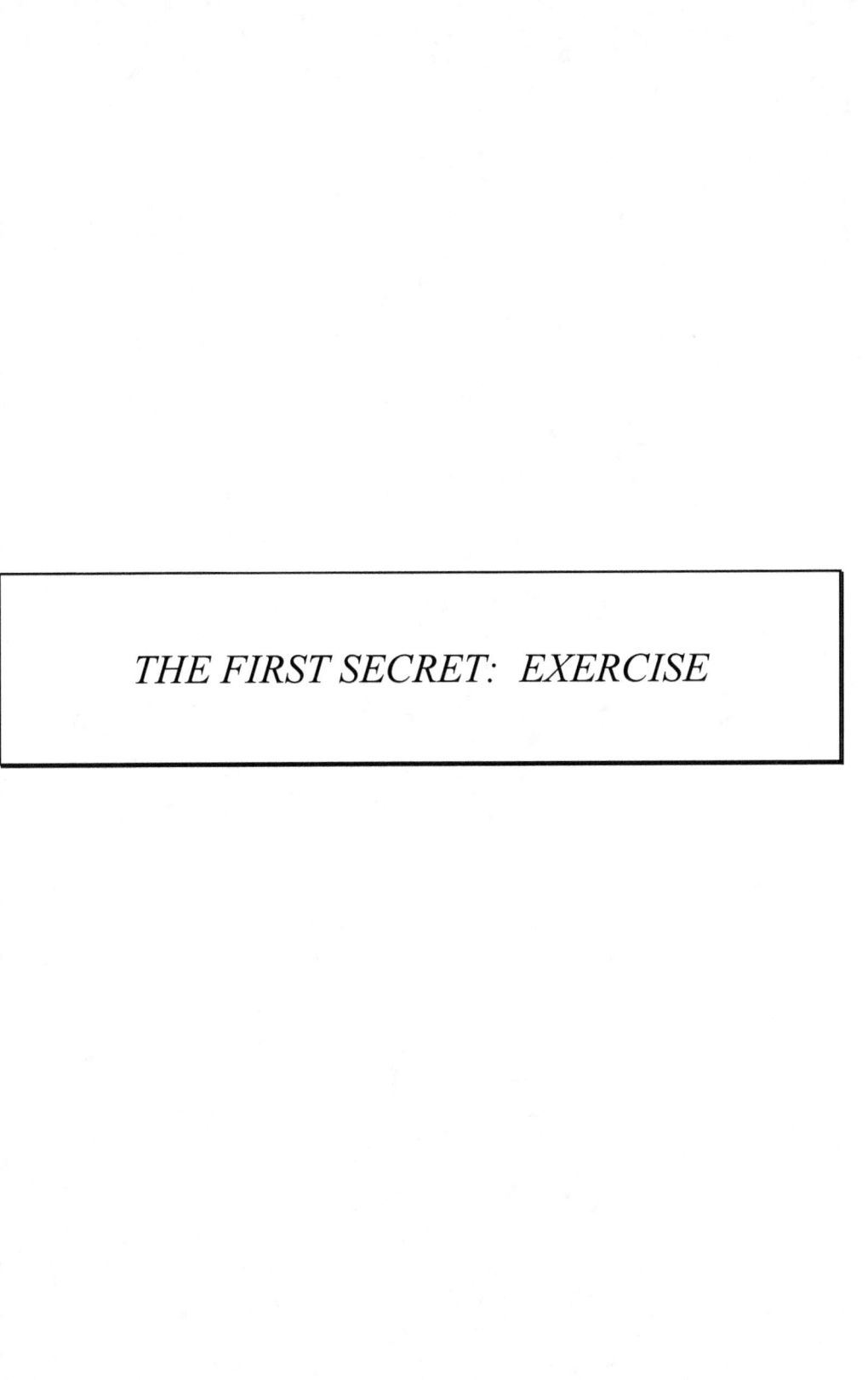

THE FIRST SECRET: EXERCISE

The First Secret: Exercise

Joan Rivers quipped, "Whenever I get the urge to exercise, I just lie down until the urge goes away." In our society, exercise is generally not held in very high regard. Sadly, our lifestyles are mostly inactive: We drive everywhere, we hold sedentary jobs, our children grow watching TV while munching on unhealthy snacks instead of running outdoors. If someone decides to take up an exercise program, it is usually part of a new diet – temporary, something that must be endured, only to be abandoned at the first sign of an achy muscle. We resent the time it takes; we rail against the sweat and the sore muscles; and we often use it as an excuse to have an extra helping at the next meal. We have not learned to value exercise for its own sake.

Humans were meant to move, and specifically to walk and run. We stand upright, and have relatively large buttock and thigh muscles. There is a reason for this architecture: It is meant to facilitate locomotion and conserve energy while chasing quarry over long distances. However, since we have made so many advancements, we no longer have to forage for our food or pursue animals for our dinners. We no longer have to till our soil to produce our food, as we did a scant 100 years ago. We now have it all handed to us: at the supermarket where food comes processed, packaged and sterile, and at restaurants where we are served portions that would feed an entire family for a week in other parts of the world. We overeat and lead sedentary lives. Exercise has been relegated to the jocks and weekend warriors.

But regular exercise - the consistent, steady movement of our bodies, is so critical to our existence, it is astounding that it does not assume a more prominent role in our lifestyles. Indeed, exercise might well be the antidote to the suffering in our society: the depression, obesity, and epidemic increase in chronic illnesses; a remedy that, rather than being a bitter pill to swallow, actually produces enormous pleasure, in addition to some compelling benefits:

- It tones the muscles
- It improves balance, strengthens your core, and promotes elimination
- It keeps the joints, ligaments and muscles supple and strong (Motion is Lotion)
- It burns calories and stokes the metabolism
- It reduces the appetite
- It improves circulation and strengthens the heart
- It improves lung capacity
- It regulates blood sugar levels
- It produces endorphins, improves mood and decreases depression
- It improves cognitive functioning
- It improves sexuality.
- Etc.

And the best exercise is ... drum roll, please ...

WALKING! Walking is a natural activity for which our bodies were well designed. We stand upright so our locomotion is accomplished with our lower limbs; we have relatively long legs, and large thighs (much to the chagrin of some). Our feet are small in relation to our entire bodies, yet contain fully one-quarter of the bones in the entire human body. A human foot is only 14-15 percent the area of the body. It has 26 bones, along with 33 joints and over 100 muscles, tendons, and ligaments. The lowly foot evolved as a platform to support the rest of the body, as well as to be able to propel the body in several directions with the action of its sinews. Such combination of mechanical attributes represents a staggering amount of raw power concentrated in one small area of the body.

It Tones the Muscles. Consider the mechanism of walking. As you ambulate, you put one foot forward, while pushing off with the other. The action of pushing off tightens all your muscles from your glutes to your hamstrings, your calves, Achilles tendon, and the plantar aspect of your foot. Most of your foot muscles and joints are activated in the movement. As you push off, that foot must sustain your entire body weight as it propels you forward before your other foot touches the ground in front of you. Your sense of balance is thus engaged.

It Improves Balance, Strengthens Your Core, and Promotes Elimination. When you walk, your arms move in counterpoint to your legs – when your right leg is forward, your left arm is back, and vice versa, so that as your legs swing, so do your arms. Auxiliary muscles are also involved, including your abdominals, which are instrumental in keeping your body upright as you walk. Your abdominal muscles are engaged as you walk, thus strengthening your core, while stimulating your digestive organs, promoting proper elimination.

It keeps the joints, ligaments and muscles supple and strong - Motion is lotion. By keeping your muscles strong and elastic, your joints and ligaments are also maintained strong and supple, which in turn help support your bones, thus reducing the risk of injury and atrophy. Exercise encourages increased range of motion of the joints (*Exercise May Ease Arthritis Pain and Stiffness*, Mayo Clinic Staff).

Motion is Lotion. One of the scourges of old age is lack of flexibility. Another is stiff joints. Yet the best way to ward off these problems is to keep yourself moving. As you move, your body produces chemicals that lubricate your joints and keep them supple. Your body creates hormones that feed your muscles and keep them strong. Arthritis is not inevitable. And the antidote is exercise.

It Burns Calories and Stokes the Metabolism. Exercise does more than burn calories; it produces a continued effect on the metabolism by boosting its performance to continue to burn calories throughout the day, hours after the initial effort (Quick).

This benefit is undoubtedly the most popular. Yes, exercise burns more calories than simply sitting at the cinema. Moreover, brisk exercise also revs up the metabolism, which helps to burn calories at a faster pace even after the exercise is finished. This may allow you to eat a bit more generously during mealtimes. And yet ...

It Reduces the Appetite. Paradoxically, vigorous exercise dampens the appetite. Contrary to popular myths, it does not increase appetite. Your body needs a period of adjustment before the hunger hormones return at full strength. Your appetite is regulated by various brain hormones that operate on a different timing and for different reasons than those that are activated during exercise. When you exercise, your body is on a kind of alert, akin to stress. That is why appetite is incompatible with the stress response. Once the stress abates, your body slowly returns to homeostasis, and hunger reappears. Of course, we have learned to override our natural hormonal ebb and flow as we have moved up the technological ladder to our current states. Because of a release of specific hormones associated with hunger, ghrelin and peptide YY, exercise also serves to decrease the appetite (ScienceDaily).

Improves Circulation and Strengthens the Heart. This dynamic movement, involving such a large number of muscles, also improves the circulatory system. As you walk, your heart rate increases, thus pumping more blood to all your organs. With heavier breathing, oxygen is absorbed into your bloodstream, oxygenating every part of your body, including your brain. The longer and more sustained your walking, the more collateral blood vessels develop, thereby decreasing the workload on your heart. It improves the cardiovascular system - Exercise delivers oxygen to the muscles; it promotes increased blood flow; it encourages the formation of capillaries, especially in the legs, serving to improve circulation; it oxygenates the lungs; it transports nutrients through the blood vessels (Sports Fitness Advisor, *The Cardiovascular System and Exercise*). And it is this same oxygenating effect that improves concentration by increasing oxygen's availability in the brain. The cardiovascular system is also responsible to a great extent for blood pressure levels. By exercising the heart muscle itself, it becomes better able to control blood pressure, which is nothing more than the pressure of the blood flow through the vessels. The stronger the muscle pumping that blood, the easier its flow. But the heart itself is only part of the story: the vessels themselves are also involved. Exercise has been shown to decrease cholesterol, thus serving to prevent or decrease the plaque that forms within vessel walls.

It Improves Lung Capacity. The lungs are living, breathing organs, full of blood vessels and capillaries. The more exercise you engage in, the better your circulation; the better your circulation, the more capillaries you will produce. And the increased capillaries will inure to your lungs' benefit as it improves your breathing capacity, protects you from asthma and other breathing-related illnesses.

35

It Regulates Blood Sugar Levels. There is a diabetes epidemic in our country. The epidemic is of such proportions, that our medical delivery system is choking. Americans spend nearly $190 billion every year on costs related directly or indirectly to obesity, according to the CDC. This is an enormous economic burden, not to mention a tragedy considering the health problems it represents, and the life-shortening implications. Obesity-related illnesses include diabetes, heart disease, cancers, hypertension, osteoarthritis, depression, and Alzheimer's, to name just a few. All these are awful illnesses in their own right, but realizing that they are all preventable is staggering. The single most important cause of these dread diseases is obesity.

Regular, sustained exercise not only serves to burn calories, but also burns blood sugar. In addition to an overabundance of processed foods, obesity has been linked to insulin resistance, where, after years of overdoing sugars and processed foods, the pancreas is no longer able to regulate its production of insulin, or the way the body uses insulin to burn blood sugar. This is where exercise is so beneficial: It adds one more layer of protection to a dysfunctional metabolism, helping to burn excess glucose in the bloodstream. Insulin is a hormone that is released by the pancreas in order to reduce the amount of sugar in the bloodstream. The liver releases glucose in response to increased demand, such as exercise. Blood sugar increases after eating – and spikes after eating simple sugars - and unless controlled, excess blood glucose becomes insulin resistant. When the body becomes resistant to insulin, this hormone can no longer effectively mop up excess glucose in the blood. This can lead to diabetes, not to mention obesity and its many associated problems. It has been shown that with moderate exercise, your muscles can take up almost 20 times the normal rate of glucose from the bloodstream, thus keeping glucose levels steady (Heath, et al).

Exercise has been linked to improved sleep, improved elimination of toxins from the bloodstream, and an improved digestive system. In fact, there are few areas which exercise does not help. And this makes sense when you consider that our ancestors lived an active life, either chasing prey over long distances, or foraging for roots. Later, we evolved to more domestic lifestyles, but it was not until the twentieth century that our society saw the shift to a monetary way of living, rather than an agrarian one, and we became increasingly sedentary. When I speak of exercise, I am referring to walking, especially outdoors. No need for an expensive gym membership, no need for colorful leotards, no need to purchase complicated equipment, no need to suffer through weeks of sore muscles in a new yoga class. Each of these has its proponents and certainly offer benefits, but for the sake of this discussion, I am referring to walking, our most natural form of locomotion, the most immediate, inexpensive and direct form of exercise, which has been shown to produce all the above-listed benefits - and more.

It Produces Endorphins, Improves Mood and Decreases Depression. Research has provided compelling evidence that exercises increases the production of endorphins, the "feel good" chemicals in the brain. That is what is colloquially referred to as "runner's high." A number of studies have shown that moderate exercise produces hormones known as neurotransmitters and endorphins, the so-called feel-good hormones (*Depression and Anxiety: Exercise Eases Symptoms*, Mayo Clinic Staff).

Posted on Facebook recently: Food is the most abused anxiety drug; exercise is the most underutilized antidepressant.

It Improves Cognitive Functioning. While we are discussing the effect of exercise on the brain, let's also remember that exercise improves concentration and cognitive abilities, including and especially memory. As discussed earlier, exercise, especially aerobic exercise, increases blood flow, which carries oxygen and nutrients to all parts of the body, including the brain. Studies have shown increase in blood volume to the hippocampus, the center of learning and memory. Improved cognition means improved memory, multitasking, and planning, and these improvements may well mean prevention of age-related decline in executive functioning.

It improves Sexuality. Exercise improves strength, muscle tone, flexibility and endurance - all critical for a healthy sex life. But there are also specific exercises, such as Kegels, to tone the pelvic muscles.

Indeed, I have found that walking produces joy and exhilaration which is enough to spur me on to continue to do it. Since I live in a warm climate, I endeavor to begin my day by taking a walk before the sun rises. This, in itself, has several benefits, not the least of which is the awakening of the body and its functions, and the ritual preparedness for the day ahead. I do not use exercise to lose weight. In fact, when I began my program of self-healing, it was because of depression, not because of overweight. I was convinced that the excess weight was a symptom of my depression and lack of self-esteem, not a disorder in and of itself. In an effort to conquer my depression, therefore, it seemed that exercise was an essential component, especially when performed

vigorously enough to take my mind off my troubles. When I take my walk, I do not listen to music on listen to audiobooks, or use earphones for any other purpose. I simply walk. I listen to the birds and to my own thoughts. I go over my day, I plan and process any troublesome areas in my life.
Typically, I will put on some comfortable clothing and go outside as part of my morning routine. I may start a bit easily, but I will push myself to get a bit out of breath. I am quite careful in this domain, however, because (1) I have asthma, and do not care to exacerbate my condition, which would defeat the purpose of getting healthy; (2) I do not wish to push myself to such a point so as to be sore the following day, get myself out of commission and unable to exercise; and (3) the objective of exercise is exercise. Period. I'm not training for a competition and am not using it as a tool for weight loss (although obviously it is a necessary tool). Simply, I exercise because it makes me feel good afterward. After 30 minutes out in nature, I am back home, I take a cool/warm shower, get dressed in clean clothes, put on some light makeup, put on some perfume, and proceed to sit at my desk, feeling invigorated, energized, clear-thinking and calm. I feel proud of myself that I overcame inertia. I feel confident. My mind works better. I remember more. My projects seem to line up easily without creating stress, and all of this is the result of oxygenating the blood, increase its circulation, so that my entire body is tingling. Incidentally, it really doesn't matter when you exercise, however, doing it in the morning has a couple of benefits: The air is clean of smog and you are setting yourself up with vibrancy to meet your day.

I remember once seeing a young woman who was considerably overweight speed-walking for exercise, in a breathless, totally unnatural pace, no doubt in an effort to speed up her results. I saw her again the next day, and again the following day, and then saw her no more. If my own experience is any indication, she probably became terribly sore by overdoing an exercise program to which she had not been prepared, but the scale had not budged an ounce. If there is a lesson to be learned here, it is that exercise really should be done for its own sake, not as a source of immediate results, as one who follows a diet: It should be a complete lifestyle, and the food should complement that lifestyle.

The word lifestyle has become a buzzword in our society, to the point that we no longer focus on its meaning: diet and exercise are a lifestyle - not a temporary endeavor to shed 50 pounds in two weeks for your sister's wedding. Take a look at your life, at the whole of your life: are you happy? Sure, you enjoy that chocolate cake, but after eating a slice, are you better off? It took you five minutes to consume that cake, and five minutes later you remain with its memory. If you have another piece of cake, it will provide similar pleasure for about five more minutes, and then what? The memory will remain. How many times will you need to remind yourself of how that cake tastes to be satisfied? So it is with other foodstuffs. The pleasure that comes from consuming them is momentary, fleeting and ultimately unsatisfying because it produces only a momentary euphoria.

Whatever results you are seeking will not happen overnight, much to our chagrin, I'm sure, and yet that knowledge should be liberating. Allow yourself to eat "enough;" allow yourself to feel richly satisfied in your new lifestyle. Discovery what makes you truly, deeply happy and pursue that. Be realistic. Don't create fantastic scenarios that are not likely to occur. To claim that the only way you could be happy is to inherit a million dollars is foolish. There are sources of happiness and satisfaction all around in everyone's life, but for many they have become obscured by other stresses.

This is the purpose of this book: to encourage you to rediscover your muses. Dare to go beyond chocolate. After all, if you are going to create a new lifestyle that is to serve you for the rest of your life, you would naturally want it to be rewarding and satisfying to go the distance. This is not a flash in the pan, so don't engage in activities which you know you cannot sustain, or activities which you know will sabotage your efforts, such as aches and pains. Be true to yourself when you assess your ability to deal with those aches and pains when they come, and adjust your activities accordingly. Do not make drudgery out of designing your new lifestyle. If you love to dance, by all means, dance! It is terrific exercise and produces even more endorphins than simply walking, because of the music involved.

Remember - exercise is one of the most critical components to a healthy lifestyle, both physically and emotionally.

The benefits of exercise are not limited to burning calories or tightening your butt. Walking is not confined to your legs only, it engages your entire body. By improving your brain function, you are also improving your sleep; by toning your muscles and strengthening your core, you are simultaneously improving your sex life; by increasing the flow of serotonin, you are averting depression and anxiety, thereby putting yourself in an enhanced condition to deal with stress, overcome life's vicissitudes, and be happier in the bargain.

Having established the merits of walking as the perfect exercise, what is the best time to exercise? Early morning. There are several reasons for that: The air is at its cleanest after a night free of traffic, and your body has just awakened from slumber, a period of hibernation, when all your bodily functions have slowed - your heartbeat, your digestion, and many of your brain functions have all have slowed down.

Sleep is a recuperative function, and when the body awakens, it is still in the grip of a slowed metabolism for some time. It is therefore essential to revive the body and bring it back to full functioning in order to deal with the stresses of life. Our ancestors slept in caves or in the open, and had to be alert to the slightest sound; we, on the other hand, no longer have to be so alert, and have therefore learned to sleep more soundly. Therefore, awakening the body becomes of vital importance in order to tackle the day's tasks with vitality. And one of the most important organs to be awakened is the brain. Walking briskly, especially outdoors, oxygenates the blood, pumps up the heart which promotes circulation all over the body, including and especially the brain.

Exercise as discussed here refers to walking. While I am not denouncing other forms of exercise, such as boxing or triathlon training, the discussion herein is geared toward those who typically shun exercise. Walking is natural, invigorating, readily available, and easily accomplished, without complicated equipment or expensive gym memberships. Moreover, you don't need to suffer through weeks of sore muscles. Walking, especially outdoors, is our most natural form of locomotion, the most immediate, inexpensive, and direct form of exercise, which has been shown to produce all the above-listed benefits - and more.

THE SECOND SECRET: AVOID TRIGGER FOODS

The Second Secret: Avoid Trigger Foods

There is no question that there are certain foods that trigger us to want more. Some of my own triggers are nuts and sweets of all kinds. There are some "experts" who advise that one should consume one's favorite foods "in moderation" - have just one or two pieces, and then stop. That's fine in theory, but in my own case, I have found it extremely difficult to control how much I consume of these foods. I don't know how to have one Pepperidge Farm cookie. I have never learned the skill of having a half cup of popcorn, or sitting down with 10 potato chips. I do know, however, how to have none, and have therefore found it easier to simply avoid these seductive morsels. Is mine the only answer? Of course not, but it eliminates the struggle. There is no conflict in my mind as to the choice I need to make – I've made it. Some people have asked me how I can watch others eat a croissant or bagel or another of my favorite foods and not indulge; how can I stand baking bread for my husband and not eat any. I liken it to being married. I may see a handsome man pass my way, I may admire him, I may even lust after him, but I choose not to act on my thoughts. There is no such thing as "irresistible."

Over the past 17 years, I have faced many occasions where lavish food was served: the week-long cruise we took through the Caribbean with the midnight "Chocolate Buffet"; the several trips we took to my homeland in Israel; various weddings, christenings and other affairs, but so far I have not indulged in what for me would be quite dangerous in terms of catapulting me right back to depression and lack of self-esteem. The temptation is quite formidable in its seductiveness: you don't go on a cruise every day; you'll get back to your program when you get home; one or two pieces will not put any weight on you; oh, come on! How could it hurt? It's a parentheses around life; don't overindulge; learn to control yourself, etc., etc. But in the end, I did not indulge. My own countering messages included: you already know the taste of chocolate; or one more piece going to make a difference? Is it going to enrich your life? How will you feel in the morning, knowing that you gave in? By abstaining, I did not feel I was depriving myself; did not feel that I was somehow missing out. There were so many other foods and experiences that I had indulged in on the cruise which I do not always do in my "normal" life: There were dancing and theater productions every evening; there were roulette tables; there were parties of every kind going on throughout the ship; the foods served were unusual, delicious and plentiful, and the shore trips were delightful, energizing and culturally diverse enough to be interesting. There was precious little that I was depriving myself from. Adding one more indulgence surely would be over the top. Besides, I already knew the taste of chocolate. I did not need confirmation.

There are no parentheses around life. If one uses the excuse of a wedding to overindulge, then what about Grandma's 85th birthday? Or the holidays - Thanksgiving, Christmas, Easter, or the Fourth of July? What about the next trip to Italy? There are innumerable excuses to overeat. Our friends' birthdays, the graduation of our children, our parents' retirement - there is no end to these so-called parentheses around life. Life is a continuum of drudgery and celebration, mourning and rejoicing. Do not delude yourself into thinking that you will count calories and shed that extra 10 pounds in the next four days. You know you will not. Experience has already taught you that. Determine here and now to use such celebrations as occasions for different forms of congratulations: a speech, or a special dress, or painting a mural as a gift.

When we went to Israel, my family prepared some of my favorite foods. My brother told me to just relax and be prepared to put on 15 pounds in the next two weeks. But at the end of the two weeks, I could have flown home with my own newly-acquired wings of victory: not only did I not gain the threatened weight, I had not indulged. The turnovers indeed beckoned, the *baklavah* was dripping with nuts and honey, my favorite sesame confections were constantly luring me, but so were other pleasures: the smell of the fig tree in our garden, the taste of fresh figs and fresh guava, the trips in the desert, the swim in the blue Mediterranean sea, the fresh sardines grilled over an open fire, the hummus and salads of every kind served at every meal, and the sharing of love and laughter and memories with my family – those honey cakes did not hold a candle to that experience!

Do I ever miss those goodies? Of course. I am bombarded by the same messages that confront everyone else. But I have come to realize that everything is a choice: to indulge in a piece of cake is a choice; to cheat is a choice; to sleep late is a choice; to watch a particular TV show is a choice; and how we react to what happens around us is a choice. Everything is a choice, and it is therefore incumbent upon us to try to make the best choices for ourselves, choices that will improve our lives, rather than diminish them. Naturally, sometimes we overindulge as a source of solace from life's stresses, but when such indulgence leaves us feeling guilty and depressed, clearly the remedy we chose was worse than what ailed us! If I am feeling stressed or upset, I know from experience that indulging in a binge will make me feel worse on the other side, and therefore I try to avoid adding mass to the original upset. I'm not always successful, though, and each time I violate this, I pay for it with worse upset. And each time, it is a lesson that has been reinforced.

Remember: don't allow temptation to win. There is a reason it's called temptation - the desire to do something wrong or unwise. Make choices that will support you. Success breeds success.

THE THIRD SECRET: REDISCOVER YOUR FAVORITE FOODS

The Third Secret: Rediscover Your Favorite Foods

When I was in the grip of my obsession with food, I would grab anything available to satisfy my cravings. Indeed, my cravings were for the quickly digested simple carbohydrate foods, the ones that would produce a quick high. Of course, by now most of you know that with a quick high, a quicker low often follows, and the cycle begins again: craving-sugar/refined carbohydrate-high-low-craving...

Simple carbohydrates are those foods that are processed and are easily converted to sugar by the body, such as white bread and all its variations, cake, cookies, candies, chips of every kind, ice cream. One problem is that these foods are so easily available everywhere, and are the subject of a constant drumbeat everywhere we turn. Recognizing their damage to our physical as well as emotional health is the first step to developing better habits, and gravitating toward better food. But "better food" is not boring food.

As a child in Israel, after-school snacks consisted of a fresh cucumber or tomato with a sprinkling of salt, or a fresh peach from my grandfather's garden. I grew up on the Mediterranean Diet, which unfortunately I had all but abandoned when we relocated to the United States. There was a special joy in harvesting what we grew and preparing meals simply from the bounty of the earth. I grew up loving guavas, figs, plums, dates, grapes and vegetables of all kinds. Grilled sardines with a tomato salad, yogurt, squash and spinach filled with eggs and cheese – those were feasts for the body and soul.

In the United States, much media attention is given to encourage people to eat their vegetables. But the suggestion to eat one's vegetables is presented in a very unappetizing manner: steaming. No wonder people avoid them! Steaming became the recipe du jour in response to the growing obesity epidemic in the United States. Steaming does preserve vitamins and minerals, but if people won't eat them, all their touted health benefits are useless. With the industry's attempts to reduce fat and salt in people's diets, it has also managed to squash any desire to eat those very foods that support good health. Enter the Mediterranean Diet, a diet rich in fruits and vegetables that are prepared to please the palate as well as support good health. The Mediterranean Diet is legendary in promoting good health, and I don't think you will find a single steamed carrot anywhere in the Middle East. So, go ahead, cook your vegetables in olive oil and garlic; add condiments like salt to your food (see my article, "The Salt Police." It's indeed ironic that in a country where obesity is at epidemic rates, fast food restaurants are on every corner, processed packaged food occupies the greatest space at most supermarkets, and people are thrown a curve ball when they are admonished to abolish sugar, salt, butter or any number of culinary additives! How can the food industry reconcile all those chemicals contained in packaged foods? Is it any wonder people remain confused about their diets?

I wrote an article called "Vegetables - a Love Affair," in which I discussed how critical the message to children should be when introducing them to good eating habits. It is sad, ironic and frankly silly to see television commercials showing people picking at some steamed broccoli with a pained look on their face, complaining that vegetables taste "too vegetably," and are therefore encouraged to get two servings of vegetables in every 8 ounces of V8 Juice. What kind of a message are you giving your children when the very mention of the word "vegetables" must be suppressed, as in the commercial for

Chef Boyardee with their slogan, "Obviously Delicious, Secretly Nutritious"? Why keep it a secret? In a recent newspaper column, there was an article entitled "10 ways to get more vegetables in your diet." Those 10 ways focused on hiding those vegetables, somehow sublimating them, disguising them. For example, they proposed making a "pasta" dish with spaghetti squash instead of noodles, or adding shredded carrots to muffins, or puree pasta sauce with vegetables such as winter squash or chopped broccoli. All this effort underscores the idea that vegetables are second-class foods that somehow must be tolerated, and if we absolutely must eat them, let's devise ways to disguise and mask them, and render them into something completely unrecognizable. How sad.

As a child in Israel, we did not have fast food restaurants, frozen dinners or Twinkies. We had a mere icebox, so nothing was frozen. My grandmother would prepare the meals daily, from fresh ingredients that she either grew in the garden or bought at the market. I consider myself fortunate to have been introduced to fresh fruit and vegetables from my earliest years in the kibbutz. Breakfasts included salads of every kind, hard-boiled or poached eggs, milk and bread. Lunches and dinners always were centered on grilled eggplant with tahini (a sesame puree), hummus (pureed chickpeas with garlic, lemon and olive oil), *labneh* (condensed yogurt), spanakopita (a Greek spinach and cheese turnover), grilled lamb or chicken skewers, and bins full of fresh figs, dates, nuts, plums and pomegranates. I am surprised how many people do not like vegetables, or have no idea how to prepare them other than steaming.

The Mediterranean Diet has been shown to be one of the healthiest, protecting against heart disease, many forms of cancer, diabetes - you name it. Yet, the Mediterranean Diet is NOT low in fat, salt, and sugar or low in taste. Indeed, the Mediterranean Diet is rich in good fats, fully flavored with salt and spices, milk and honey from the land. Find your bliss here. See how you can recover your taste buds. Do not deprive yourself of an essential joy in life. Find out how to nourish your body as well as your soul.

I write a blog called The Food of The Mediterranean where I share some of my favorite recipes, but Israel is a melting pot of many cultures, all of which have had their influence on the food. There are people from Greece and Turkey, Morocco, Tunisia, Eastern Europe, Ethiopia, to name a few. All of them have contributed to the food of Israel, which is really the food of the Mediterranean.

Everyone has his or her own favorite foods that represent fond memories, foods that are healthful and nourishing to both body and soul. The challenge is to reacquaint yourself with those memories and reintroduce them into your life.

Remember: do not allow yourself to be deprived. Eating a boring plate of steamed cauliflower will not satisfy your soul, will not abate your hunger, and will not help in the long run. Do not substitute one obsession for another, from the obsession with fast, easy food to an obsession with the last diet or an obsession with exercise. Take the time to learn how to prepare delicious food that is life sustaining. Revisit your childhood, if necessary, and rediscover your favorite foods. If those were not compatible with your current thinking, make the effort to learn about the Mediterranean Diet. There is no "rabbit food" in the Mediterranean Diet: the food is rich in flavor, fully satisfying, nourishing and healthful, and deserves to be a prominent component of a healthy lifestyle.

THE FOURTH SECRET: LIFE'S OTHER PLEASURES

The Fourth Secret: Life's Other Pleasures

I have already alluded to some of my other pleasures in life beside food. There are so many, in fact, that it is astounding how easily they become relegated to second and third place in favor of food. I might even state that there are several pleasurable activities, which surpass the pleasure that food provides.

For example, earlier I spoke of exercise. Granted that some effort is involved in stepping outside in the morning. But the coolness of the morning air cannot be underestimated in the pleasurable sensation on one's skin. For that matter, the way I feel when I am done, after my shower, when I am ready for my day's work, cannot be duplicated by a Danish. It is a delicious feeling to be clean and cool and fresh and energized. Not to mention proud of oneself.

I am fortunate in that close to my home is a large lake. Typically mornings bring flocks of birds of all kinds to the lake in search of food or mate, and the chirping and whistling is music to my ears, as is the sheer beauty of seeing them in flight, reflected in the water.

Speaking of music, I love classical music and jazz. I have some favorite composers. Preparing my meals with the sounds of Kathleen Battle in the background is heaven on earth. Sitting quietly while listening to Rachmaninoff is equally exhilarating, while the sophisticated lyrics of Cole Porter inspire me to write poetry.

The first cup of coffee in the morning is a cherished practice for me. Since I rise early, the house is still quiet, and I am free to be with my thoughts as I sip the hot, fragrant brew, preparing to take my walk.

As mentioned earlier, my walk itself is pleasurable as I make my way around the lake, and that pleasure is magnified by the cool shower I take upon my return. Spraying some light perfume tops the experience.

When I lived in Miami, Sunday mornings would be reserved for the beach. I would arise at dawn, and find the beach cool and deserted, with the only sounds being the squawking gulls and the rush of low tide breaking the silence. That was my paradise.

Remember - life is full of pleasures beyond food. Discover your own.

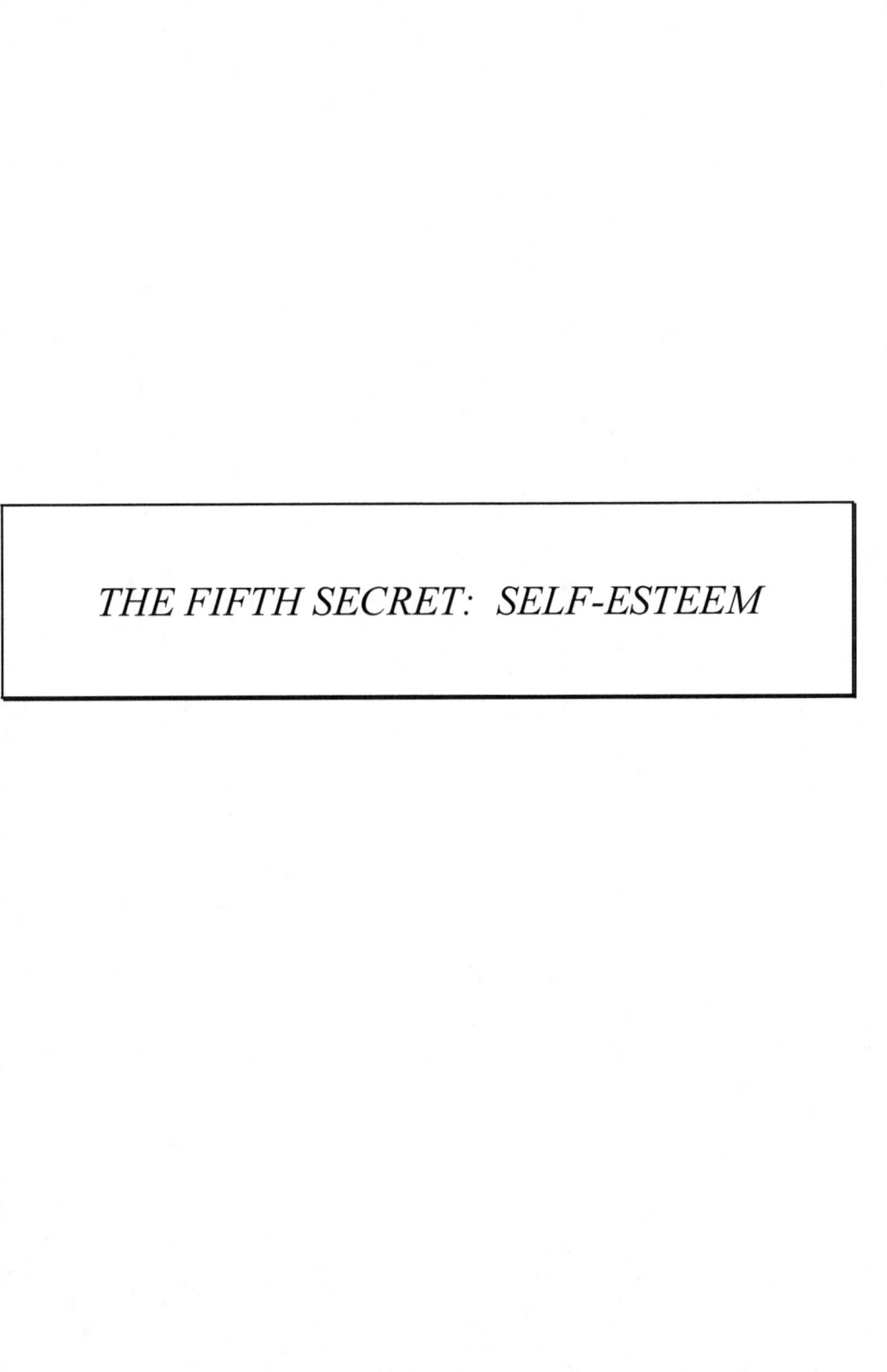

THE FIFTH SECRET: SELF-ESTEEM

The Fifth Secret: Self-Esteem

To improve self-esteem, do "esteemable" things. In its simplest form this means do those things, which will increase your pride in a job well done. Do not avoid what is difficult - tackle it. Face your fears. Attack your challenges. One of the greatest self-esteem builders is courage. Courage does not mean not being afraid -- it means acknowledging the fear and doing it anyway. Face your dragons. Lend a helping hand, even if you don't want to -- especially if you don't want to. Do your exercise because you gave your word, even if you don't feel like it. Hold your tongue instead of lashing out automatically. In other words, whatever you do which enhances your sense of pride in your behavior and actions also enhances your self-esteem. And increased self-esteem means increased self-confidence, the trust that you can face the challenges of the world, that you can tackle any task and not cringe. And *nothing* feels as good as self-confidence. A feeling of self-confidence is far reaching in its benefits. It gives you a sense of being unshakable, of being competent, of being able. Self-confidence comes the self-knowledge that your word is your bond, your word is good, you are trustworthy; if you give your word in any endeavor, you can be trusted to keep it and follow through. This is true even if others do not recognize it. Your sense of self-confidence rests upon you, on your word -- not what others may perceive. Being trustworthy is a gift you give yourself. It is a measure of your strength that you are ready to step up, that you will not cower. The recovering alcoholic can take a drink in hiding, and no one will know, but he will; and that act alone will shatter his self-esteem. Honor is a character trait that distinguishes you as a generous, giving individual, rather than someone who tries to get away with anything possible in order to further his or her own agenda or avoid pain.

With some minor modifications, the following is an article I published some time ago:

I failed BASIC

When I was in college, I was a very good student, but it came at a deep price. I was obsessed with studying, driven with doing a good job, to the point that I was deeply anxious almost all the time. The anxiety kept me up nights, ruminating and mentally mapping all my potential strategies for the next thesis or the next test. The reports I wrote were produced after hours spent in the library doing research, poring over many books, taking profuse notes, frequently staying until the wee hours of the morning, writing, copying, reading. The results were wonderful, but I was a wreck. Test taking, by contrast, was hell. My anxiety level was so high, I suffered from severe migraines. In fact, in the case of the final exam in computer programming, I was so anxious that I completely blanked out after writing my name on the test paper! Blanked out. Nothing, nada, zip. Not even reading through the multiple-choice answers jogged my memory. I handed in my blank test in defeat, hearing the dreaded words from the teacher, "You're going to fail the course, you know." Yes, I knew. And I did.

Computer programming was not a required course for graduation, so I allowed that F to fester on my transcript. I ignored it. I made excuses for it. I didn't talk about it. The years passed, and somehow I made good in my other courses, until the time came to apply for graduation. However, it appeared that although I had completed my required courses, my elective courses, as well as several graduate level courses, there was an entry-level course that was required which I somehow had not fulfilled. I could not graduate

without it. Bummer! That is when the offending F
from computer programming came back to haunt me.

It seemed totally pointless to take only one 101 course
for three months on my way to graduation. I talked
about my silly predicament with my mentor/best
friend, who by now knew about my computer
programming fiasco/F on my transcript. He suggested
that I take two classes: The missing required course
AND the computer programming course. What?!?
OMG. The old anxiety came in again like a tsunami,
forceful waves washing over me, angst, dark memories
about blanking out at the final exam! After much hand
wringing, I said I would do it. I gave him my word
that I would not quit, no matter what. Even if it meant
another failure, I would not quit. My butt would be in
that class for every session, I would pay attention,
would do the assignments, I would go the distance.

Do you know how it feels to have just given your word
about something so scary? You might as well have
extracted a promise from me that I'd walk on fire! No
matter what, I'd go the distance?!? What, are you
nuts? Don't you know I have no head for computers?
I don't need this class anyway, it's not a required
course for my major, it was an elective in the first
place!

After all this hand-wringing, I stepped over to the other
side. The side of resolve, serene acceptance, of
surrender. There is a wonderful poem by Goethe:
"Until one is committed, there is all manner of
hesitancy, …"

I signed up for computer programming, the same
course I had previously failed. My professor this time
was a colorful, muscular, gorgeous specimen of a

human being, with a crinkle in his eye and an attitude of taking no prisoners. He had no sympathy. He raked everyone over the coals, and when I presented one of my papers "backwards" in the sense that I first wrote out the steps, and then drew the flowchart, he announced in front of the whole class that "you will bomb the test." OMG! I knew enough about self-fulfilling prophecy to really worry about that, so I meekly replied, "Don't bet on it." That drew some groans of respect from my fellow classmates. I was intent on defeating whatever pronouncements were out there in the universe intent on sabotaging me.

It was Thanksgiving week, and we had one month to complete our class project. The final exam was scheduled for the end of December. His words rang loudly in the crevices of my mind, and I did not feel my retort was nearly as powerful as his prophecy, but I had given my word to Woody, and I was committed. I could not back out.

Thanksgiving Day, 10 a.m., I showed up at the university computer lab, project in hand. In those days, if you got up from your assigned computer and someone else sat there, you were out of luck, and had to wait your turn again. I was assigned a computer and began to collect my thoughts. Again, I preferred to write my steps down, and then proceed to do the flowchart. I had designed the project with a few shorthand notes, and then proceeded to translate it onto a computer program. It was an airlines reservations motif with seat assignments and meal preferences. Reams and reams of printed paper later, I was done. The program flowed nicely, all the loose ends tied in a bow. It was 11 p.m.

I presented my finished project to the colorful professor in class Monday. He leafed through it, reviewed my precepts, reviewed the flow of information, and declared, "This is beautiful. You don't have to take the test." What? I was excused from the final exam, the monster that had haunted my dreams, the ogre that had tormented my sleep?

V-I-C-T-O-R-Y!

THAT is self-esteem.

Nothing - not chocolate, ice cream, diamonds or sex could improve on that feeling of accomplishment.

When I claim that my self-esteem was enhanced by these actions, I am not being conceited; this is no holier-than-thou proclamation. Rather, it is that I feel better about myself as a consequence. This is not self-righteousness. It is self-appreciation.

Is this easy? No. But it is this very challenge that reveals your mettle. Most people have to work for a living, but would not keep their jobs if they only went in to work when they felt like it. Children would not be cared for if parents only got up when they felt like it. Most people drive, and do so by following the rules of the road. They do not get to vote on whether they like those rules – they already did. If you want to drive, you also accept the responsibility of following traffic laws. So it is with your self-esteem. Being trustworthy is an asset. Being trustworthy means you can be relied upon. Giving your word is a responsibility. It follows you around. You are not required to make a promise or a commitment, but if you do, your self-esteem rests on keeping your word.

Remember - to build self-esteem, do "esteemable" things.

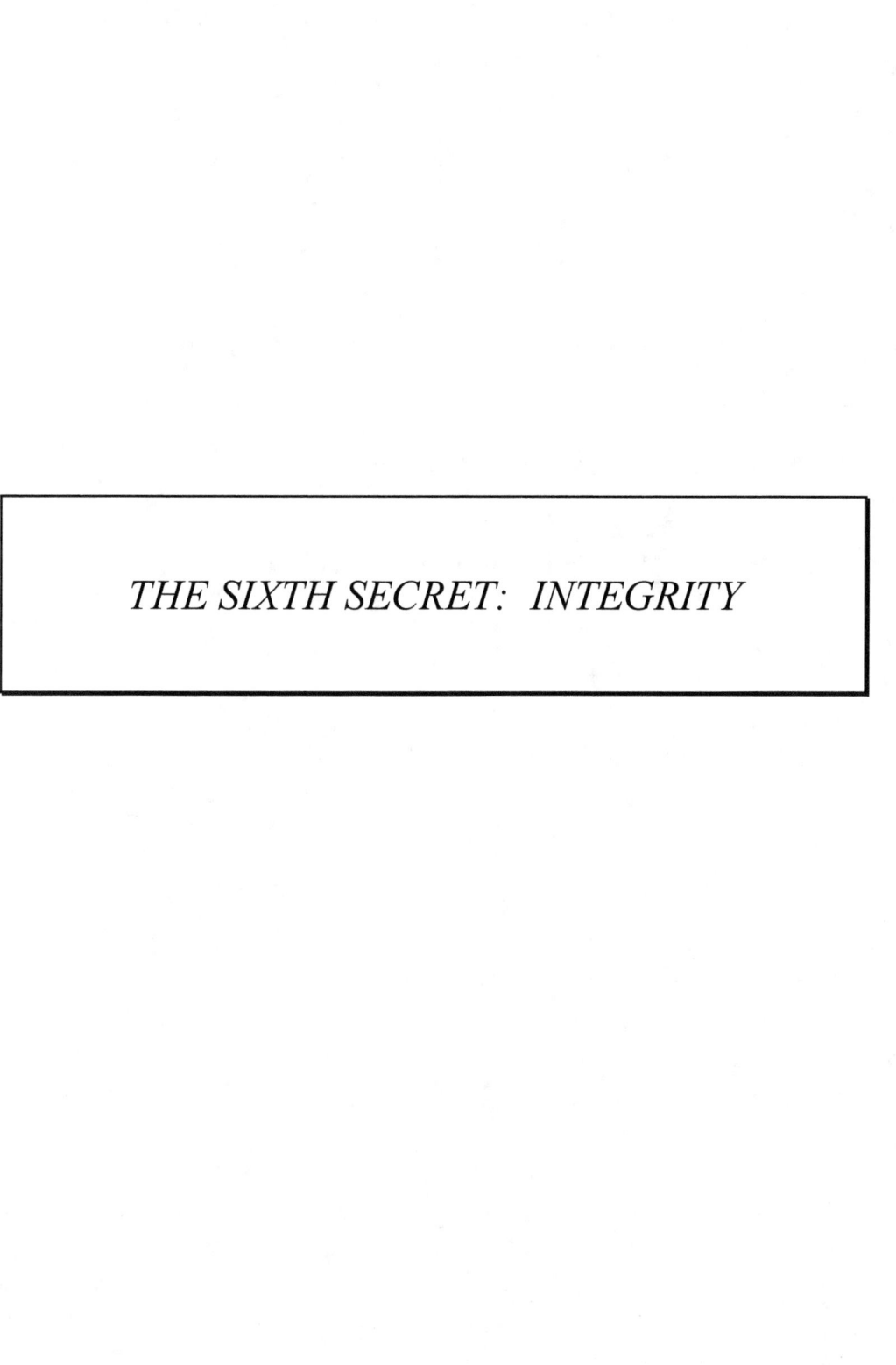

THE SIXTH SECRET: INTEGRITY

The Sixth Secret: Integrity

What is integrity? Integrity is honesty, truthfulness, honor, reliability and uprightness. It means being true to yourself, honoring who you are fundamentally. It means being reliable to keep your word. This is not some airy-fairy admonishment being handed down at the pulpit - integrity affects and shapes your life. Living with integrity has little to do with "proving" that you are telling the truth. Living with integrity is for your own sake. Living with integrity eliminates internal conflict. There is no push and pull over decisions. Integrity refers to moral fiber, inner strength, and determination. It is your character, your temperament and disposition. It speaks of your principles and values, what is important to you and how do you go about defending it. If the next promotion is important to you, how do you go about getting it - by backstabbing your colleagues, or by doing your best to merit it? And if you are passed over, how do you deal with it - with poise and equanimity, or with a jealous, vindictive rage?

Living with integrity means living authentically. Do not hurt yourself or others, not even in jest. Indeed, realize that by hurting others, you are in fact, doing harm to yourself. Be quick to make right any misunderstanding. Be quick to forgive, to let go of a grudge. Do not speak crossly to others, and do not self-deprecate. There is enormous power in the spoken word. Don't indulge in complaints and bitterness. Try to eliminate them as much as possible, in favor of more positive talk.

While some of this might sound suspiciously like preaching, I assure you it is not. Studies have shown that the words we speak and the actions we take shape our lives and our thoughts. Cognitive psychotherapy maintains that simply behaving a certain way shapes our thoughts, which in turn shape our feelings. I have included some references in the bibliography of books written about virtue. One such seminal work is the *Book of Virtues* by William Bennett. Both virtue and sin play into the concept of integrity.

Remember - qualities such as loyalty, commitment, courage, and forbearance are traits that can be cultivated to further your own health.

THE SEVENTH SECRET:
GRATITUDE

The Seventh Secret: Gratitude

Spiritual groups abound, from candle vigils, prayer meetings, and Twelve-Step programs. People everywhere are turning to a Higher Power. In each case, this Higher Power is called upon as a source of help and the object of gratitude. No matter what one's personal circumstances, gratitude should be paramount in one's mind. We are truly fortunate to be free to choose our lives, we should be thankful for all we have: our health, the food we eat, whatever pleasures we experience, as well as our challenges. It is our challenges that build our character and test our mettle. Even difficulties and tragedies can be sources of gratitude when looked at in a new light. Give thanks for the friends you have and the people who care about you. Give thanks for living in a country where clean water runs freely. Give thanks for the sunshine, and your ability to see the sun. Give thanks for your work. Give thanks for your talents. Give thanks for a moment's quiet. Give thanks for your children, and all that they teach you. Give thanks for your parents and all they have taught you. Give thanks for your favorite teacher. Give thanks for your successes and your failures, and give thanks for the lessons learned from them. Give thanks for who you are. Be open to new experiences. Be quiet in your soul. Be good to yourself.

Thank you for taking this journey with me.

THE DIET-PROOF LIFESTYLE

- ➢ The Mediterranean Diet
- ➢ Memories of a Bygone Era
- ➢ What Can I Eat On The Mediterranean Diet?
- ➢ Samples of Mediterranean Classics

The Mediterranean Diet

Throughout this book, I have attempted to discuss the causes of obesity, along with its many terrible consequences. I am not overstating it when I say that our entire economy would flourish and thrive if by some miracle we were able to reverse our obesity rates. I have already demonstrated that we consume much of our food in processed form, with added colorings, excess salt, sugar and fat. We have become accustomed to shopping for boxed or canned or preserved foods, with little regard to quality. Even those of us who read labels are not immune from this calamity. We have come to accept nutrients described in the form of chemicals on labels. We have been educated to shun certain manufactured oils as detrimental to our health, but we have not crossed back over to a more natural diet. Indeed, our government has attempted many times to reverse the trend of obesity by introducing low-fat or low-sugar consumables, only to cause even greater weight increases and disease. All the fat-free and sugar-free campaigns have done more harm than good. According to some reports (Aubrey), we are fatter now than before the fat-free boom.

We have come to rely far too much on processed foods. It is no secret that Americans love meat, especially red meat, and that our diet as a whole has become inordinately adulterated from its natural state. The chart below shows the percentage of calories we consume from whole as compared to processed foods:

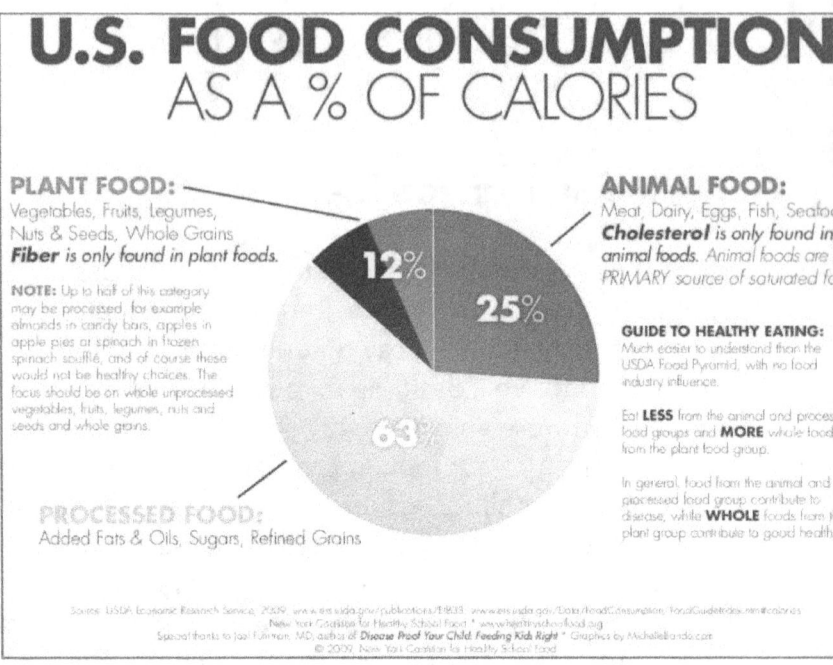

U.S. FOOD CONSUMPTION
AS A % OF CALORIES

PLANT FOOD:
Vegetables, Fruits, Legumes,
Nuts & Seeds, Whole Grains
Fiber is only found in plant foods.

NOTE: Up to half of this category
may be processed, for example
almonds in candy bars, apples in
apple pies or spinach in frozen
spinach soufflé, and of course these
would not be healthy choices. The
focus should be on whole unprocessed
vegetables, fruits, legumes, nuts and
seeds and whole grains.

ANIMAL FOOD:
Meat, Dairy, Eggs, Fish, Seafood
Cholesterol is only found in
animal foods. Animal foods are the
PRIMARY source of saturated fat.

GUIDE TO HEALTHY EATING:
Much easier to understand than the
USDA Food Pyramid, with no food
industry influence.

Eat **LESS** from the animal and processed
food groups and **MORE** whole foods
from the plant food group.

In general, food from the animal and
processed food group contribute to
disease, while **WHOLE** foods from the
plant group contribute to good health.

12%
25%
63%

PROCESSED FOOD:
Added Fats & Oils, Sugars, Refined Grains

Sources: USDA Economic Research Service, 2009, www.ers.usda.gov/publications/EB33, www.ers.usda.gov/Data/FoodConsumption/FoodGuideIndex.htm#calories
New York Coalition for Healthy School Food * www.healthyschoolfood.org
Special thanks to Joel Fuhrman, MD, author of *Disease Proof Your Child, Feeding Kids Right* * Graphics by Michelle Bonde.com
© 2009, New York Coalition for Healthy School Food

You will note at a glance that 63 percent of our food
consumption is in the form of processed foods, and a mere 12
percent plant food! In fact, it is astonishing that many people
consider French fries a vegetable!

This book promotes the Mediterranean Diet, which is rich in
fruits and vegetables, grains and nuts, as well as the bounty
of the sea. The Mediterranean Diet is legendary in promoting
good health, and is as varied as it is full of flavor. I do not
believe you will find a single steamed carrot anywhere
throughout the Middle East. This diet includes healthy fats
that serve to satisfy hunger, along with all known spices and
herbs that make a cuisine palatable.

So go ahead, cook your vegetables in olive oil and garlic; add
condiments like salt to your food (see my article, *The Salt
Police*). It is indeed ironic that in a country where obesity and
its accompanying degenerative diseases are at epidemic

rates, fast food restaurants are on every corner, processed packaged food is the most plentiful at grocery stores, while we are simultaneously thrown a curve ball when we are admonished to abolish sugar, salt, butter, and any number of culinary additives! How is the food industry reconciling the artificial chemicals contained in packaged foods? Is it any wonder people remain confused about their diets?

After some experimenting, you may find that you can eat to your heart's content and stop micromanaging sugar grams or calories, exchange points or hours at the gym.

Memories of a Bygone Era

This is not a cookbook, nor is it a diet book. It is a repository of my memories of childhood in Israel, the sights, sounds and smells of Israel, and the feelings they evoked then as well as now. As a child, I relished my grandmother's cooking, and the special confections she prepared, like the *bourrekas* and *sharope, kadaiff* and *baklava*. Inevitably, some of my favorite recipes will be featured, and I will also intersperse updated recipes of renowned chefs from around the world.

When I was a child, we lived in a small village with unpaved roads. We had no television sets, and many families had nothing more than an icebox. One of my fondest memories of childhood is my grandmother's daily walks up to the main road where the ice man would lead a donkey with a cart full of large chunks of ice, which he would cut and lay a piece on a cloth on my grandmother's shoulder. One day, he arrived as usual, but the donkey was accompanied by her baby, a fluffy miniature that delighted all the neighborhood children.

I wrote an article called Vegetables – a Love Affair (see Appendix) in which I discussed how critical the message to children should be when introducing them to good eating habits. As a child in Israel, we did not have fast food restaurants, frozen dinners or Twinkies. We had a mere icebox, so nothing was frozen. My grandmother would prepare the meals daily, from fresh ingredients which she either grew in the garden or bought at the market. I consider myself very fortunate to have been introduced to fresh fruits and vegetables from my earliest years in the kibbutz, and I lament how many people I meet who do not like vegetables, and would never consider eating a whole fruit as a snack.

The Mediterranean Diet has been shown to be one of the healthiest, protecting against heart disease, many forms of cancer, diabetes - you name it. Yet, the Mediterranean Diet is NOT low in fat, salt, sugar, and certainly not low in taste. Indeed, the Mediterranean Diet is rich in good fats, robust flavors, seasoned generously with salt and spices, milk and honey. Find your bliss here. See how you can recover your taste buds. Do not deprive yourself of an essential joy in life. Find out how to nourish your body as well as your soul.

I write a blog named, The Food of the Mediterranean, where I examine the many cultures that have emigrated to Israel, all of which have brought their country's culinary practices and recipes to the region. There are people from Greece and Turkey, Morocco, Tunisia, Eastern Europe, Ethiopia, to name a few. All of them have contributed to the food of Israel, which is really the food of the Mediterranean. The people who emigrated to Israel over the years were of varying ideologies, but many of them came to a country prepared to work the land. In the early years of its existence, Israel was largely agricultural, so food was fresh from the land, and was prepared in the styles of all the peoples and countries represented. It was the agricultural background of Israel that supported the plethora of vegetable dishes of every kind that the Mediterranean diet's renowned healthfulness is known for Mediterranean Diet.

Nowadays, I have a slightly different, more inclusive, philosophy. Since my husband is Japanese, I have naturally been influenced by the cuisine of the Orient. That region of the world follows a diet rich in fish, but is also a cornucopia of vegetables, fruits, nuts and spices. In many ways, the cuisine of the Orient resembles that of the Mediterranean, with small differences in cooking methods, spices and herbs. There are some foods which seem ubiquitous throughout the world, like rice, for example, which graces the dinner plates in the Orient as in the Mediterranean. Lentils, spinach, eggplant, salads of every kind adorn the tables of almost all cultures in the world. There is such variety, and it is so well prepared and so tasty, I cannot imagine vegetables not appealing to the taste buds of just about everyone. Yet, in the United States, vegetables are rarely given such a lofty position in our culinary arsenal. Indeed, what passes for vegetables is invariably either steamed without flavoring, or worse, as French fries.

America was built on the backs of the pioneers. To be sure, food was scarce, but the bounty of the land was available and celebrated as a feast at Thanksgiving. The wild turkey, corn and sweet potatoes would be welcome on any Mediterranean table. The Pilgrims came from impoverished England and Ireland, where their diet consisted mostly of lamb and potatoes. They arrived in New England where they remained poor for years, then the wagon train took many pioneers across a land inhabited. On their journey, they subsisted on cured bacon, beans and meat from their cattle. This country was built by pioneers with an eye toward independence from religious oppression. The American Indians, for their part, grew corn and hunted turkeys and buffalo, ate sweet potatoes and tomatoes, and supplemented their diets with some nuts and fruit, but theirs was a diet limited to what they could find or grow locally. The gold rush miners came next, and their lives were characterized by shanty towns with muddy roads. Their focus was on striking it rich, not on cultivating the land.

Because of the influx of Chinese immigrants who worked on the early railroads, Chinese and other Oriental cuisines began to be introduced to the American palate. Today, we find Korean, Japanese, Indian and Thai cuisines interspersed among their American counterparts to seduce us with their fare. These Oriental cuisines make heavy use of vegetables and spices to appeal to the palates of its consumers, and are as healthy as they are delicious. They have become ubiquitous alternatives to the traditional American diet.

The cornerstone of the Mediterranean diet is that it is composed of fresh foods, natural foods: produce from the farms, fruit from the trees, and fish from the sea. If you wish to get away from processed foods, then stop reading labels. Buy food in its natural state.

What Can I Eat On The Mediterranean Diet?

I promise – no rabbit food!

Take a look at a typical Mediterranean diet pyramid pictured below.

Do the images look like rabbit food? No! But, you may protest, these are pretty pictures, but how do I incorporate.

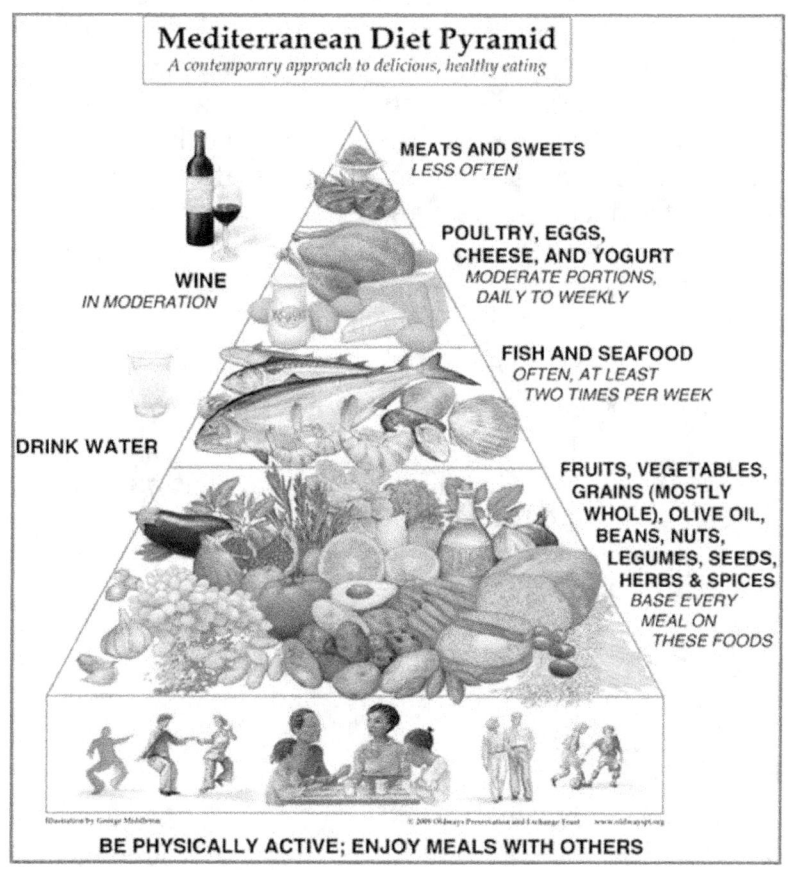

Mediterranean Diet Pyramid

A contemporary approach to delicious, healthy eating

MEATS AND SWEETS
LESS OFTEN

POULTRY, EGGS,
CHEESE, AND YOGURT
MODERATE PORTIONS,
DAILY TO WEEKLY

WINE
IN MODERATION

FISH AND SEAFOOD
OFTEN, AT LEAST
TWO TIMES PER WEEK

DRINK WATER

FRUITS, VEGETABLES,
GRAINS (MOSTLY
WHOLE), OLIVE OIL,
BEANS, NUTS,
LEGUMES, SEEDS,
HERBS & SPICES
BASE EVERY
MEAL ON
THESE FOODS

BE PHYSICALLY ACTIVE; ENJOY MEALS WITH OTHERS

Courtesy of Oldwayspt.org

these foods into my diet? A grapefruit is "diet" food, and I'll be hungry! I'm not suggesting that you restrict your diet.

Indeed, this entire book is about enjoying your food to the fullest, relishing every bite, reveling in the fact that you are honoring the temple that is your body and nurturing good health.

The Mediterranean Diet emphasizes the gamut of plant-based foods, from vegetables, roots, nuts, herbs, seeds and fruit, to the grains, including breads, rice, pasta, couscous, and any combination thereof. The pyramid is constructed in such a way as to display the greatest emphasis in the diet, and curiously, at the bottom of the pyramid, the widest part, are images of people being active. That is the most prominent aspect of the Mediterranean lifestyle. Above that are the staple plant-based foods that are the cornerstone of the diet; above them, in ever-decreasing segments, are the seafood, poultry, eggs, yogurt and dairy foods, with meats and sweets occupying the uppermost segment of the pyramid, indicating their ingestion to be at the lowest frequency. Wine in moderation, and water is to be drunk liberally.

Samples of Mediterranean Classics

In a future book, I shall describe the many possible recipes that can be prepared with Mediterranean fare, and shall focus on the simplest recipes to prepare. For now, let's look at some of the available delicacies that you might enjoy:

Breakfast:
- Banana pancakes with slivered almonds and honey
- Vegetable omelet with tomato, onion, dill and feta cheese
- Potato and tomato scramble
- Bowl of amaranth cereal topped with yogurt and honey
- Lemon turnovers
- Coffee cake with strawberries and guava
- Turnovers with cinnamon, cardamon and cream cheese
- Buttered poppy seed cake
- Leek and goat cheese fritata
- …and many more!

Lunch:

- Savory fava beans with warm pita bread and tahini
- Roast eggplant stuffed with chicken and tomato
- Roast zucchini, summer or winter, sautéed with tomato, garlic and onion served over rice
- Chicken at la Turque served with sweet potatoes, onions, and apricots
- Pasta salad
- Tuna salad
- Halibut sandwiches on crusty bread

Dinner:

- Mediterranean lamb cooked with mint and apricots
- Chicken roasted with garlic cloves and lemons, served with potatoes
- Potato casserole with chopped lamb and tomato
-         Lamb kebab with bloody Mary sauce
- Seafood grill with scordalia
- Chickpea patties (falafel) stuffed into hot pita bread with tahini, cucumbers and tomato
- Babaganough and hummus
- Portobello mushrooms stuffed with meat and garlic
- …and many more!

My purpose here is to introduce you to the richness that is available on the Mediterranean diet. Please note that none of the above is prepared with ersatz cream or butter, but with the real thing! No artificial this or fake that; no sugar substitutes or margarine. Each one of the above dishes is delectable and healthy. What is missing from the above list are the deserts, of course. Trust me when I tell you that nothing can compare to a good *baklavah*, although admittedly, I recommend indulging in this delicacy sparingly.

As for drinks, they run the gamut from plain refreshing water to mint tea, either hot or cold, as well as rich dark coffee as drunk in the Mediterranean region.

To your health!

EPILOGUE: A NEW BEGINNING

EPILOGUE: A NEW BEGINNING

You have read the book, pondered on some of the ideas promoted herein, and hopefully you feel inspired. Now is a time to take stock, evaluate what you've learned, and examine what fits and makes sense. Begin to think of how you will incorporate changes into your daily life. This is the time to adapt and adopt a new lifestyle, without entirely abandoning your old one. Look again at the elements that contribute to a life well lived. We talked about secrets that appear outside mere attempts at weight loss. We talked about some profound concepts that are useful guideposts on your journey. We discussed various diets, the effect of dieting on your brain, calorie counting, the diabetes epidemic worldwide, the obesity epidemic and its contributors. We then explored some values that have stood the test of time for millennia, and which are solid beacons on the road to success. The seven secrets of success are:

1. Exercise
2. Avoiding Trigger Foods
3. Rediscovering Your Favorite Foods
4. Life's Other Pleasures
5. Self-Esteem
6. Integrity
7. Gratitude

To be sure, there are more. One essential secret not listed above, but discussed previously, is enjoying a plant-based diet, rich in polyunsaturated oils and omega-3 fats. We discussed the merits of the Mediterranean diet. Diet proofing your life is all about balance, small steps, and looking beyond the superficial effects of a instant gratification and keeping our eye on life's other pleasures.

APPENDIX

Supplemental Articles
By the Author

- ➢ The Salt Police
- ➢ Vegetables – A Love Affair
- ➢ Physical Fitness – The Missing Link
- ➢ Water
- ➢ The Trouble With Sugar

The Salt Police

There was an insert inside the latest edition of Prevention Magazine promoting their latest book, The Salt Solution, which was being billed as the best way to shed pounds, protect your life, keep you young, indeed, increase your bank account -- you name it, they promised it, if you would only give up salt! And they were not talking about merely eschewing the salt shaker -- they were talking about hidden salt that seems to lurk at every turn, devilishly intent on causing us harm.

It cited studies that have shown improved sleep, improved concentration, improved disposition and improved sex. High blood pressure, diabetes, heart disease, cancer and obesity have all been shown to be related to excess salt in the diet. They cited the proliferation of processed foods in our diets, restaurant foods with hidden salt, and salt hiding in many unexpected places, with the result that we are consuming far too much salt in our diets.

I have not conducted any scientific research. And I respectfully defer to the scientists who have. I do not question that too much salt contributes to hypertension and other ills, and that learning how to modify our diet is advisable.

I have stopped eating in Italian restaurants. Although I lived for a short time in Italy and love Italian food, the American version of Italian food is insipid by comparison. Every recipe for pasta calls for salt in the cooking water. Cooking shows abound on TV, and each program shows the host adding salt to the water. And yet in Italian restaurants, the pasta that is served is bland, tasting like cardboard with red stuff on top. Restaurant chefs seem to think that drowning pasta in marinara sauce will somehow imbue it with flavor. It does not. I had the "pleasure" of ordering pasta y faggioli soup at a rather high-class bistro recently, and was served a garlicky mélange of something inedible, because it had no salt.

Salt is one of the most ubiquitous flavor enhancer. It is one of the cheapest, most abundant condiments. Salt is a preservative. And we all need salt in our diets. Having said that, there is no doubt that many people overeat salt, be it from potato chips to popcorn, pizza or Nachos, there is no doubt that salt is pervasive in our diets. But so are butter and beer, coffee and cigarettes. So are corn syrup and monosodium glutamate. So is a host of other chemicals, preservatives and hydrogenated fats. My objection is not to the message that we must reduce salt in our diets. Perhaps it's true. My objection is to companies taking it upon themselves to police my consumption. In the bistro that served the insipid pasta y fagioli soup, I remarked to the server that the soup needed salt (there was no shaker at the table), to which he answered, "Salt isn't good for you." Really!? But there are other items on the menu which are equally "not good for you," including steak and duck, and some rather decadent desserts dripping with butter, chocolate, whipped cream and sugar. In fact, there was a container of sugar and Sweet 'N Low at the table! Where do you draw the line? Obesity and its side effects have been linked to our sedentary lifestyle, as much as our overconsumption of processed foods. But this is a philosophical matter, one which should focus on educating society in better lifestyles, not policing their choices.

A friend once gave a speech that began, "Who Wants to be a Millionnaire?" The whole room enthusiastically raised their hands at the prospect of some new bit of information that would improve their lives. No, this friend promptly produced a pack of cigarettes, and enjoined the group to smoke until they became sick, and then sue the tobacco companies. That was tongue in cheek, of course, but the message was clear: You cannot eschew the choices that you make. And so it should be with food. To be sure, as with cigarettes, studies have shown that the fast food companies are counting on the addictive qualities of some of their offerings in capturing their audiences, and keeping them coming back for more, thus escalating the battle of the bulge. But there is a question of contributing negligence here. We as a society have choices to make, and claiming that a substance is addictive is not an excuse.

About 30 years ago, the government got into the act of trying to reduce sugar in the diet. It mandated that food companies begin a systemic reconfiguring of their recipes, including posting detailed labels of the grams of sugars present per serving. The effect was that those companies simply found ways around the new mandates: They began substituting cane sugar with sugar substitutes, as well as increased fats. The end result was that statistically, we are far heavier now than we were before such laws were passed.

As it was with the Prohibition, when government regulation prohibited the selling of spirits, so it is in so many ways now that the tentacles of government are trying to control our lives in many subtle, and not-so-subtle ways. I say enough. If you feel you need to reduce your salt (or sugar or fat or what have you) intake, by all means, go for it. Education is a much better form of power, education both at the school level, as in the media, as in the home. If you want to learn to love vegetables, learn to prepare them in appetizing ways. If you want your children to be healthier and more energetic, don't fall for the easy way out. We all have choices, and ultimately the power is in our hands.

Vegetables – a Love Affair

Yet another newspaper article has been written, this time by Jennifer Larue Huget, extolling the virtues of green vegetables. She repeats the tried-and-true information that we all know - or should know - that vegetables are great sources of vitamins and minerals, are typically low in calories and are a great source of fiber. She cites two experts in the field, Alexandra Postman, editor in chief of Martha Stewart's Whole Living magazine, and an editor of "Power Foods" cookbook, and Jim White, spokesman for the American Dietetic Association. She then proceeds to list five vegetables that top the list in nutrients and other good-for-you characteristics, but again, like so many others, states that "steaming is the best way to retain nutrients." Other vegetables that made her list include spinach, artichokes, asparagus and celery. As for celery, she gives as a tip to "use celery as a 'vehicle' for healthful toppings such as almond butter, peanut butter..." She proceeds to list the calories per cup as 16 (but NOT if they are used as a vehicle for anything!)

It is stunning that such articles are written in the first place. Is it possible that Americans don't know that vegetables are healthy? that vegetables have vitamins, minerals and fiber? No. Americans already know that. The problem is that vegetables are not made palatable in the United States. Vegetables assume second-class status to cheeseburgers and foot-long hot dogs and French fries. In fact, in a recent episode of Man vs. Food, a show that features the most obscene quantities of heart and artery-clogging ingredients, one of the commercials was for V8 juice, which was touted as tasting just like fruit juice for those who think "vegetables taste too vegetably." Are you kidding me? Taste too vegetably? And to juxtapose that commercial within a show of unabashed gluttony is misplaced, to say the least. How is the industry ever hoping to reeducate people into better eating habits? In fact, even the idea of presenting vegetables disguised in a fruit juice is absurd.

Enter well-meaning writers such as Jennifer Larue Huget. Her intentions seem lofty enough. But her message is distorting. In her article, she features broccoli as being one of the best vegetables around, listing its many credentials; but she ends her segment with a tip that "steaming is the best way to retain [broccoli]'s nutrients." I agree, and would go a step further by stating that eating it raw straight from the garden would be even more healthful. The problem is not her assertions - it is that people do not like steamed vegetables of any kind, and do not eat them. And broccoli seems to be at the top of the list. Why perpetuate an idea that people will not follow?

I have long maintained an affinity for the Mediterranean diet. I have written loudly about it. I have written that from my earliest years, the diet of my country consisted of all forms of vegetables, all either cooked and well seasoned or made into colorful salads with lovely Mediterranean dressings. In fact, I assert that nowhere in the Middle East will one ever find a steamed broccoli flowerette.

The point is not that steaming is not good; it is. But if it does not inspire people to eat the vegetable, what's the point? Indeed, it is like recommending to a hungry man to drink a glass of water! It will not satisfy, and if something does not satisfy, it is not likely to be repeated. All the tips and information about vitamins and minerals, fiber and cancer-obliterating miraculous foods are meaningless if people will not avail themselves of them. And pointing out that celery is a vehicle for almond butter, and then claiming that one cup has only 16 calories is a ridiculous contradiction.

In the past 100 years, we have come from a mostly agrarian society to a society that thinks deep-fried Twinkies are essential for good health or that French fries constitute a vegetable. There seems to be so much confusion, that articles are written about real food. How do we turn back the clock? The emphasis should be placed on teaching people that "real" food can be palatable, indeed, delicious. Sautéed spinach in a bit of olive oil with some minced garlic and sliced onion would add tremendous flavor and few calories, and will also be relished and probably become a favorite menu item.

Physical Fitness - The Missing Link

Fitness means readiness. Being fit means being well (healthy), able-bodied, ready to participate fully with life and deal with the environment and its various challenges. Fitness refers to the overall condition of the entire body: the physical, the mental, and the emotional. All of these components are interconnected, working together, to accomplish the complex requirements of living.

We all want more energy – energy that lasts all day; vigor to carry us through our daily chores; mental agility and alertness to facilitate our tasks; and the vitality that accompanies good health. For many people, these are indeed high aspirations. Unfortunately, they are also elusive. We have become far too sedentary, victims to technological advances.

Yet it is not technology that is the villain, but rather how we have adapted to technological advances. For example, in the field of nutrition, each time the food industry has introduced a new-fangled product to help us shed excess pounds – artificial sweeteners, low-fat products, sugar-free products, etc. – we have gotten fatter. Since 1962, for example, the obesity rate in the United States has gone from 13 percent to a whopping 39 percent by 2010. That is astonishing, and quite alarming.

Technology has also been instrumental in automating many of the chores we used to perform manually. Instead of mopping the floors, we now have RoboVacs. Instead of chopping, mincing, and sautéing, we now "set it and forget it." Instead of playing sports, we play video games. Our lives have become a series of push-button conveniences. And where these so-called conveniences are supposed to support our lives and make us more productive, they have in many ways proved deleterious to our overall health.

How do we design our lives in such a way as to counter the effects of so much inactivity? Must we eschew our washing machines, spend a fortune to join a gym, or buy the latest leotards? No. We can continue to enjoy our convenience toys, the latest gadgets, and our cars, while still engaging in some essential physical exercise that is both enjoyable and free.

The next best exercise is dancing.

That is why we have muscles and movable joints. If we were meant to be inactive, our anatomy would be completely different, to conform with our needs. If our needs only involved pushing buttons, our entire physiology would morph. If science fiction is any indication, we might one day all develop into the likes of Barbarella, and do everything electronically!

But that day is not yet upon us. We are not mental beings. And until such time as we are able to overcome our physicality, it is incumbent upon us all to heed the alarms being sounded and protect our health. We must move our bodies.

Paradoxically a singular reason why people take up exercise: they want to lose weight. They think that the calories contained in the pizza they had for lunch will be wiped out with an hour's run. Under the best of circumstances, an hour's run would only burn about 400 calories, while that pizza lunch probably amounted to 2000 calories, or more.

Water

Life would not be possible without it. Our bodies are made up of approximately 60 percent water. Life began in the ocean; embryos are nurtured in a water environment; even NASA has sent up Discovery to search for water on Mars as a sign of possible life.

Water is essential to life: Why do we need water? Water is essential to carry nutrients to various parts of our bodies, for the metabolism of food and to carry toxins out of the body. And for healthy hydration, a body needs a constant replenishment of water. This is accomplished by drinking water. Water is lost from various functions of our bodies, not the least of which is sweat. If we do not supplement it, we become dehydrated, which leads to fatigue and muscle cramps, as the body is not receiving proper nutrients.

Water to stay slim: Water is also essential to stay slim. An obese person has less water as a percentage of body weight than does a slim person, as lean tissue and muscle contain more water than adipose tissue.

Types of water: The types of water that are commonly available include tap water and bottled water. Some adventuresome types might drink rain water or spring water, but for the more urbane among us, bottled water is considered the safest, cleanest water. The bottling process undergoes various stages of purification of the water from chemicals, such as chloride and lead, which also contributes to the taste of water being sweeter and more palatable.

How to increase consumption: It has been determined by scientific research that a human being needs approximately eight glasses of water per day, sometimes

102

more as in hot climates or if doing strenuous exercise. But many people resist drinking so much water, preferring to drink alcohol or sodas, neither of which replenishes the body with what it needs to function. Drinking eight glasses of water is relatively easy, if one begins the day with a glass of water, has another glass at midmorning, then another with lunch, two in the afternoon and one with dinner. Water can also be taken in teas, and if one is a fan, there certainly are enough varieties on the market.

Simply knowing that sweet-tasting, pure water is essential for health and a slim, trim body is enough of an impetus to take up the habit. And after a while, one begins to depend on the cool, delightful feeling of a glass of water.

The Trouble with Sugar

Halloween is upon us. The reason for this bacchanal has largely been lost on the majority of celebrants. Halloween marks the eve of All Saints Day, a day of remembrance of the dead, the saintly, martyred, and faithful departed believers. Halloween was designed as a way to use humor and ridicule to flout Death.

But how did an attempt to scorn Death come to involve so much sugar?!

A bit of history: Some scholars maintain that Halloween is a Christianized feast with pagan roots, perhaps influenced by European harvest festivals.

In an attempt perhaps to cheat Death, pranks, games and scary stories evolved. The Christian tradition encouraged abstinence from meat in favor of vegetarian dishes on this vigil day, along with attendance at church services and cemeteries to remember the dearly departed. In time, however, such restrictions devolved into much more commercialized festivities, with an enormous focus on sugary treats.

So what's wrong with that? It's fun, the kids love it, it's just one day a year – what's the harm? The harm is that it is not, in fact, just one day a year; sugar consumption is ubiquitous in our present-day society, much to the detriment of the population. Let's take a look at how sugar became so endemic.

The Industrial Revolution brought with it many technological innovations that helped folks move from the farm to the cities. Along with such innovations came the ability to process food on an industrial level, making many foods heretofore scarce much more easily available to the general population. Such staples as sugar, coffee, and flour could easily be mass produced. Moreover, sugar was found to be a great preserver. Our staple grains could now be processed by machines into very fine white flours, a process previously done by hand. Increasingly, society wanted to enjoy the fruits of these innovations, and it became fashionable to bake little white sugar cakes to be served on special occasions. Indeed, it was a mark of the higher ranks of society to be able to afford white flour.

The food industry – or more to the point, the sugar industry, became enormously influential in the halls of government, and in time, almost all foodstuffs became loaded with added sugar, both to extend shelf life, as well as to feed the growing demands of the population. In time, more and more sugar in all its iterations, came to appear in our food. According to the USDA, soft drink production has risen from 100 (12 ounce) cans per person in 1947 to 400 in 2000! And this is just soft drinks!

But none of this limited history lesson addresses the issue of what's wrong with sugar? Why should we not simply enjoy its delectable taste?

The answer is not a simple one.

Sugar comes in many forms, from the white table sugar we are all familiar with, to molasses, corn syrup, honey, turbinado, fructose, dextrose, maltose, sucralose, and many other variations on that theme. To know whether there is sugar in any form added to a product, find the suffix "ose" in the ingredient list. Each form of sugar plays a different role in its assimilation by the body, and there is convincing evidence that none of them is healthy. In fact, the human body needs a certain amount of sugar to function optimally. The problem is when there is an excess of this element – and our current diet certainly contains an excess of sugar. Sugar, in one of its many forms, is found in almost every food item found in the store, except foods found in the produce department. Sugar is used as a preservative; it is used to increase palatability; it is used to intensify its addictive quality; it is used to pacify babies; it is used to enhance breads and sauces; and of course, it is in just about every conceivable form of dessert, cake, ice cream or candy.

Here's the simple answer: Everything you eat is fuel for the body. Some fuel is meant to burn slowly, some fuel burns more quickly, supplying immediate energy. Simple sugars – such as candies and ice cream – burn very quickly; in other words, they are said to metabolize rapidly. It is the function of the pancreas to secrete insulin to absorb sugar in your blood stream. Whatever you eat breaks down into some form of sugar for fuel, which is then metabolized by insulin and travels through the body to supply energy to the various muscles, nerves, bloodstream, bones, etc. Any excess sugar is mopped up by the insulin secreted by the pancreas and stored in the liver. There is a certain homeostasis in healthy individuals, where the pancreas is able to produce sufficient insulin to absorb excess sugar, so that some excess sugar is not deleterious to one's health. However, that state can change with excess supplies. When there is an overabundance of that chemical – sugar – for an extended period of time, the pancreas has to work overtime to mop up that excess sugar. In time, such overwork can cause it to fail. If the pancreas fails to produce sufficient insulin, excess sugar remains in the bloodstream and you have the beginnings of diabetes.

Diabetes has become epidemic in the United States. This is not some medical term relegated to the annals of doctors' offices, for which you are simply prescribed medication that you can take while you continue your damaging eating habits. Diabetes is serious business! More to the point, it is a serious illness. It can cause blindness, peripheral neuropathy (loss of sensitivity in the limbs), gangrene, amputations, heart problems, hearing problems, blood pressure problems, and even death.

While diabetes has become epidemic, a more immediate problem with over-consumption of sugar are tooth decay and obesity. Our children now suffer the highest incidence of obesity in the world; obesity also contributes to lack of mobility which in turn produces lack of fitness. Add to that tooth decay, and the cycle of human deterioration begins to loom very large simply as a consequence of eating too much sugar, more precisely refined sugar.

What is refined sugar? It is any sugar that has been processed from its natural source. Fruits contain natural sugar, as do beets and sugar cane. If one consumes fruit in their natural state, one is consuming a source of sugar that is wholesome and complex and requires energy for the body to process. When sugar is processed into its simple components, it becomes a substance that acts almost like a drug on the body, becoming addictive and encouraging increasing amounts to satisfy that sweet tooth. It is a vicious cycle.

Sugar is essential for good health. But the kind of sugar that promotes good health is the kind that is found in the produce department – fresh fruits and vegetables, or any food that does not require a label.

Bibliography

Aubrey, Allison. "Why We Got Fatter During The Fat-Free Boom." March 28, 2014. Accessed October 25, 2015. http://www.npr.org/sections/thesalt/2014/03/28/29533257 6/why-we-got-fatter-during-the-fat-free-food-boom.

Bennett, William J. *The Book of Virtues*. New York: Simon & Schuster, Inc. 1993. Print.

"The Cardiovascular System and Exercise." http://www.sport-fitness-advisor.com/cardiovascular-system-and-exercise.html.

Cawley, J, and C Meyerhoefer. "Medical Care Costs of Obesity: An Instrumental Variables Approach." *J Health Econ*. 2012; 31:219-30. Accessed October 23, 2015.

"Depression and Anxiety: Exercise Eases Symptoms." Accessed October 23, 2015. http://www.mayoclinic.org/diseases-conditions/depression/in-depth/depression-and-exercise/art-20046495.

"Exercise Suppresses Appetite." *ScienceDaily*. December 19, 2008. Accessed October 23, 2015. http://www.sciencedaily.com/releases/2008/12/0812110814 46.htm.

Heath, G W., and J R. Gavin, 3rd. "The Effects of Exercise." August 1, 1983. Accessed October 23, 2015. http://jap.physiology.org/content/55/2/512.short.

Murray, William H. In The Scottish Himalayan Expedition,. 1951.

"Obesity Consequences - The High Cost of Excess Weight." *Harvard T.H. Chan School of Public Health*. Accessed October 25, 2015. http://www.hsph.harvard.edu/obesity-prevention-source/obesity-consequences/.

Pianin, Eric, and Brianna Ehley. "Budget Busting U.S. Obesity Costs Climb Past $300 Billion A Year." *The Fiscal Times*. June 19, 2014. Accessed October 24, 2015. http://www.thefiscaltimes.com/Articles/2014/06/19/Budget-Busting-US-Obesity-Costs-Climb-Past-300-Billion-Year.

Quick, David. "Exercise Can Stoke Metabolism." *The Post & Courier*. August 24, 2010. Accessed October 23, 2015. http://www.postandcourier.com/article/20100824/ARCHIVES/308249928.

Somer, Elizabeth, M.A., R.D. and Snyderman, Nancy. *Food and Mood, The Complete Guide to Eating Well and Feeling Your Best, 2nd ed*. New York: Holt, 1999. Print.

Withrow, D, and D A. Alter. *"The Economic Burden of Obesity Worldwide: a systematic review of the direct costs of obesity." Obes Rev*. 2010. DOI: 10.111/j.1467-789X.2009.0072.x. Accessed October 23, 2015.

Suggested Reading

American Academy of Orthopedic Surgeons, (Sept. 2009), *Exercise and Bone and Joint Conditions,* http://orthoinfo.aaos.org/topic.cfm?topic=a00100

Freedman, Lisa, (n.d.), *Can Exercise Help Curb Your Appetite?,* http://www.mensfitness.com/nutrition/what-to-eat/can-exercise-help-curb-your-appetite

Fries, Wendy C. (n.d.), *Exercises for Better Sex*, WebMD, http://men.webmd.com/features/exercises-better-sex

Hellmich, Nanci (9/8/2011), USA Today, People who exercise vigorously get a bonus for their hard work: They continue to burn extra calories long after they're finished working out, a new study shows, http://yourlife.usatoday.com/fitness-food/exercise/story/2011-09-01/Bonus-for-exercisers-Calories-burn-long-after-workout/50224116/1

Hyman, Mark, MD. The Blood Sugar Solution: The UltraHealthy Program for Losing Weight, Preventing Disease, and Feeling Great Now! 28 Feb 2012.

Lovett, Kate (n.d.), *Exercise and Disease Prevention,* http://www.vanderbilt.edu/AnS/psychology/health_psychology/exercise.htm, Vanderbilt University

McArdle, William D., BS M.Ed, Ph.D., *Exercise Physiology: Nutrition, Energy, and Human Performance* (Point (Lippincott Williams and Wilkins)), Nov. 13, 2009

Mayo Foundation for Medical Education and Research (Jan 1, 2010), *The Mayo Clinic Diet*: *Eat Well, Enjoy Life, Lose Weight.*

Mayo Clinic Staff, (n.d.), *Depression and Anxiety: Exercises Eases Symptoms,*
http://www.mayoclinic.com/health/depression-and-exercise/MH00043/NSECTIONGROUP=2

McGraw, Phil, Ph.D., "The Ultimate Weight Solution," The Free Press, New York 2003.

Myers, Jonathan C., Ph.D. (n.d.), *Exercise and Cardiovascular Health,* http://circ.ahajournals.org/content/107/1/e2.full, American Heart Association

Sears, Barry, Ph.D. with Bill Lawren. *Enter The Zone: A Dietary Road Map.* New York: ReganBooks. 1995. Print.

Smith, Allen (Oct. 27, 2009), *Effects of Exercise on Blood Glucose,* http://www.livestrong.com/article/19126-effects-exercise-blood-glucose/

Snyder, Aaron, The New Diabetes Prescription Revolution, Nov. 10, 2010

Stainback, Raymond F. (11/9/2008), *How Does Exercise Affect the Circulatory System?*
http://www.texasheart.org/HIC/HeartDoctor/answer_66.cfm

www.ingramcontent.com/pod-product-compliance
Lightning Source LLC
Chambersburg PA
CBHW071155280526
45787CB00002B/514